The Herb Book

Mary Ann Dykes

A Guide for the more serious student.
*W*ith over 50 herb illustrations.

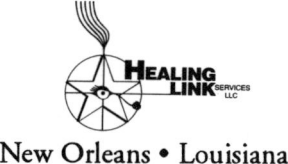

HEALING LINK SERVICES LLC

New Orleans • Louisiana

The Herb Book

HealingLink Services, L.L.C.
4621 S. Johnson Street
New Orleans, LA 70125
Published 1996

Herb illustrations by Jodi McDaniel

ISBN 0-9651890-0-7   Printed in U.S. A.

CONTENTS

*I*LLUSTRATIONS

Introduction

This book is written as a practical and simple history of herbs and herbal uses. Balance of the body is obtained not only through a single approach of natural health care such as the uses of herbs in natural healing, but also through a daily vigilance to better understand mind, body and soul. Care of the whole being - physically, mentally, emotionally and spiritually - can bring about balance and harmony to a person where there once was none.

Holistically speaking, to bring about balance we must begin with all levels of existence simultaneously.

Prevention is synonymous with vigilance. Responding to the human need to be nurtured on emotional and mental levels as well as nourished on a physical level, we maintain balance with our inner and outer environments.

And it is through this special care given the whole self, our soul, that we become able to care for others.

Open your hearts to the Earth and welcome her plants as you would a teacher.

This book provides knowledge lost to most of us in a modern society. Read and Remember.

With Warmest Regards and Blessings
Mary Ann Dykes

Warning To The Reader

This book has been written in an attempt to help recall the history of herbs and their uses and perhaps to offer education.

Neither the author nor the publisher of this book is a medical doctor and neither do they hold themselves out to be part of the medical profession or system.

Professional medical advise is recommended by the author and publisher for medical problems.

This book is not intended for people who wish to diagnose disease nor does it dispense medical advise or offer treatment for disease.

The author and publisher assume no responsibility for use of herbs or any remedies listed in this book without prior professional medical advice.

Preface

This book is a compilation of early herbal remedies, some of which are still used in our modern society.

Historically, herbs were used to act in four different ways to bring about balance.

Herbs have been used to:

1. *Stimulate*
2. *Sedate*
3. *Eliminate*
4. *Build*

The Early Chinese, the Native American, the Ancient Egyptian and the East Indian have provided records concerning the discovery of herbal uses since the beginning of time.

Early Herbology

Early Herbology was recorded first in the written record of the Sumerians dating back 5000 years ago. Early man learned from nature that herbs and plants were to be used to treat or remedy illness. Through instinct and experience herbs were integrated as a natural substance providing poisonous effects to draw out unwanted blocks in the body or to add nutrients to nourish the body. Herbs were used to soothe or to irritate -- all in an effort to eliminate or add to the body's resources. Modern day medicines originally were organic compounds found growing in nearby fields, valleys, or in wooded areas where the disease it remedied was most apt to be found.

The Early Chinese produced an herbal guide listing 365 plants including Ma-Huang. Ma-Huang was the basis for modern day ephedrine, and is still used as an alternative to synthetic drugs to stimulate the adrenals.

Hippocrates, the father of modern medicine, advocated

the use of a few herbs, fresh air, rest and proper diet. This is in keeping with a natural healing approach to imbalances. The natural life force of the body is kept in balance by the elemental forces, the play of our inner and outer environment, and the mental and spiritual effects of these forces on our sense of well-being.

The early Christian Church discouraged the practice of medicine. The intention of this was to follow the teachings of Jesus Christ which were understood to be Faith Healing; healing without the use of physical substance.

The Christian Church of the time believed that true Christianity depended only on Faith Healing, even though Christ was mentioned in the Bible as using herbs for cleansing and healing.

There was a strong need to control the masses, and in particular the peasants who relied on herbs and old methods of healing passed on from person to person. The early Christian Church advocated suppression of herbalists and pagan healers to promote one authority over Spiritual and Healing matters. That authority was the Church Fathers.

The Monasteries became the "keepers" of the herbal knowledge. They preserved and protected manuscripts concerning knowledge of herbs and natural medicine. The monasteries of the Christian Church became centers where herbs were stored and this was referred to as the "officina."

The Middle Ages brought about some of the bad feelings relating to natural healing. This was a time when witch burnings were a frequent occurrence. Because black magic and witches were thought to be connected to herbs and potions gathered by women and pagans, people burnings were held to rid the villages of "unsafe practice." This was in the 13th and 14th Centuries.

By the late 15th Century the First English Herbal was published. After that Nicolas Culpeper, MD published his book: The Complete Herbal in 1649.

In America in the 19th Century, American Folk Medicine developed as a blend of American, Indian and European Herbs. Dr. Samuel Thompson was the most outstanding exponent. Thompson suffered at the hands of medical doctors, being criticized and even jailed for his system of herbology. The Thompsonian System is still in use today.

In Germany, Homeopathic Medicine was begun and developed by Dr. Samuel Hahneman in the late 18th Century. As evidence of the origins of modern day medicine it should be pointed out that a large number of Western Allopathic Medicines, including Digitalis from Foxglove and Aspirin from Willow, are medicines originating from natural medicines.

Homeopathic Medicine, as opposed to Allopathic Medicine is developed on the premise that "like cures like." Hahneman believed that disease was a necessary part of elimination. He believed that by taking small doses of a substance that caused symptoms like the disease, a person could be cured of those symptoms.

Of course the word here "symptom" is of great importance because we understand in natural healing the emphasis is put on the whole process to reach the deeper internal as well as the external symptoms.

Nevertheless Hahneman used the like cures as well as the "minimum dose" for cure.

The premise of the minimum dose is that the body's own natural energy response to the herb that produces the symptoms to the disease will be activated. The natural forces will kill or fight off what caused the disease to begin with.

Herbs have been known as natural healers since primitive man stumbled out of the cave onto the first plant to cure his indigestion, or to help stimulate his liver as a Spring Tonic.

Herbs can act as a stimulant or sedative; or herbs can be used to eliminate toxins from the body; or herbs can build strength and nutrition for the body.

Herb Properties

Herbal Medicine uses words to describe the action an herb will have on the body. Several of these actions are listed below.

Abortifacient

An herb has this property when it will expel a fetus prematurely.

Acrid

This property of an herb would cause heat and irritation when applied to the skin.

Alterative

Gradually, the benefit of this herb would be felt and create a nutritive change in the body. This would not come about abruptly or through a specific action. These herbs are known as blood purifiers.

Analgesic

This herb would have an effect on the body that would diminish pain without causing a loss of consciousness.

Anaphrodisiac

This herb is the antithesis of an Aphrodisiac. The property or characteristic use of this herb is to reduce sexual desire or potency.

Anesthetic

This herb deadens sensation.

Anodyne

An herb that soothes or relieves pain would have this property.

Anthelmintic

This herb would cause intestinal worms to be dispelled.

Antibiotic

This herb destroys micro-organisms, such as bacteria, viruses, or amoebas.

Anticatarrhals

These herbs break up and eliminate mucus.

Anticoagulant

An herb that prevents clotting in a liquid such as blood would have this property.

Antiemetic

This herb relieves vomiting and stops nausea.

Antiseptic

This herb destroys putrefied bacteria.

Antispasmodic

This herb has properties that will stop cramps and spasms. These herbs cause the body muscles to relax and to provide energy for healing.

Aperient

This herb is used to stimulate the bowels and is a mild purgative.

Aphrodisiac

This herb has properties to increase sexual potency.

Appetizer

This herb has properties that can be used to stimulate

the appetite or the desire to eat.

Aromatic

The herb that has this property is able to bring with it an attractive and stimulating odor.

Astringent

This herb has properties that contract organic tissue, consequently reducing secretions or discharges.

Balsam

This herb is a soothing and healing herb with a resinous substance gathered from several trees to be used medicinally.

Bitter

This property or characteristic of an herb specifically acts on the mouth and stomach. This will increase appetite and promote digestion.

Calmative

Herbs with this property offer a mild sedative action on the body and act as a tranquilizer to the nerves.

Cardiac

This herb will have a direct effect on the heart.

Carminative

This herb expels gas from the intestines.

Cathartic

This herb will have an action of causing the bowels to evacuate.

Caustic

This substance will burn away tissue.

Cholagogue

This herb carries properties that will increase the flow of bile to promote elimination.

Coagulent

This herb has properties that have been known to produce clotting in the blood.

Counterirritant

This is known to produce irritation in one part of the body that will counteract a known irritation in another part of the body.

Demulcent

Mucous membranes are soothed by this herb, as it works to soothe irritated tissue.

Deodorant

This herb destroys or masks odors or smells.

Depressant

This herb will lessen nervousness or any activity. It has the opposite effect of a stimulating herb.

Diaphoretic

This herb can be used to promote perspiration.

Digestive

Properties of this herb will promote digestion.

Diuretic

These herbs increase the flow of urine. They are specifically used to reduce water retention.

Emetic

This herb will cause vomiting.

Emmenagogue

The menses will be brought on by the properties of this herb. Abortion can also be brought about through these herbs.

Emollient

This herb is used to soften and soothe.

Errhine

This herb promotes sneezing.

Euphoriant

This herb promotes unusual buoyancy.

Expectorant

This herb has the properties to bring about discharge of the mucus from the respiratory channels, specifically the lungs and throat.

Febrifuge

This herb stops or lessens fever.

Galactagogue

This herb will increase secretion of milk in nursing mothers.

Hallucinogen

This herb has properties that will bring on hallucinations.

Hemostatic

This herb has properties that will stop bleeding.

Hepatic

This herb acts on the liver.

Hydragogue

The properties of this herb will produce a watery discharge.

Hypnotic

This herb brings on sleep.

Irritant

This herb will cause inflammation.

Laxative

This herb brings about evacuation of the bowels.

Mucilaginous

A gelatinous consistency gives this herb properties for a salve or being made into an ointment.

Narcotic

This herb will relieve pain and bring about sleep.

*CAUTION: In doses to excess this herb could cause convulsions, coma and death.

Nauseant

This herb will cause vomiting.

Nervine

Known to be an herb that is nutritive to the nerves, a nervine soothes and acts on the entire nervous system.

Parasiticides

This herb destroys parasites in the digestive tract. They can also act directly on the skin.

Purgative

This herb will promote strong bowel elimination.

Refrigerant

This herb will reduce body heat well below normal.

Restorative

This herb is an agent that restores consciousness or normal activity.

Rubefacient

This herb has a gentle action of irritation and will redden the skin due to increased blood flow. The purpose is to draw inflammation from other parts of the body.

Sedative

This herb has properties that are soothing and lessen nervousness or worry. They include nervines and anti-spasmodics.

Sialagogue

This herb will increase the production of saliva. This is used to stimulate digestion of starches.

Stimulant

This herb has properties that increase activity and physical processes. They will increase the energy of the body through an increase in circulation.

Stomachic

This herb will stimulate, strengthen or bring tone to the stomach.

Styptic

This herb is an astringent, which means it will stop bleeding through contraction.

Sudorific

This herb promotes perspiration.

Tonic

This herb strengthens and brings vitality to the body.

Vasoconstrictor

This property of the herb narrows the blood vessels causing blood pressure to increase.

Vasodilator

This herb increases the size of the blood vessels, lowering blood pressure.

Vermicide

This herb has properties that destroy worms of the intestines.

Vermifuge

This herb expels intestinal worms.

Vesicant

This herb has irritating properties that produce blisters.

Vulnerary

This herb will encourage healing of wounds, internally and externally. This property works particularly on cell growth leading to repair.

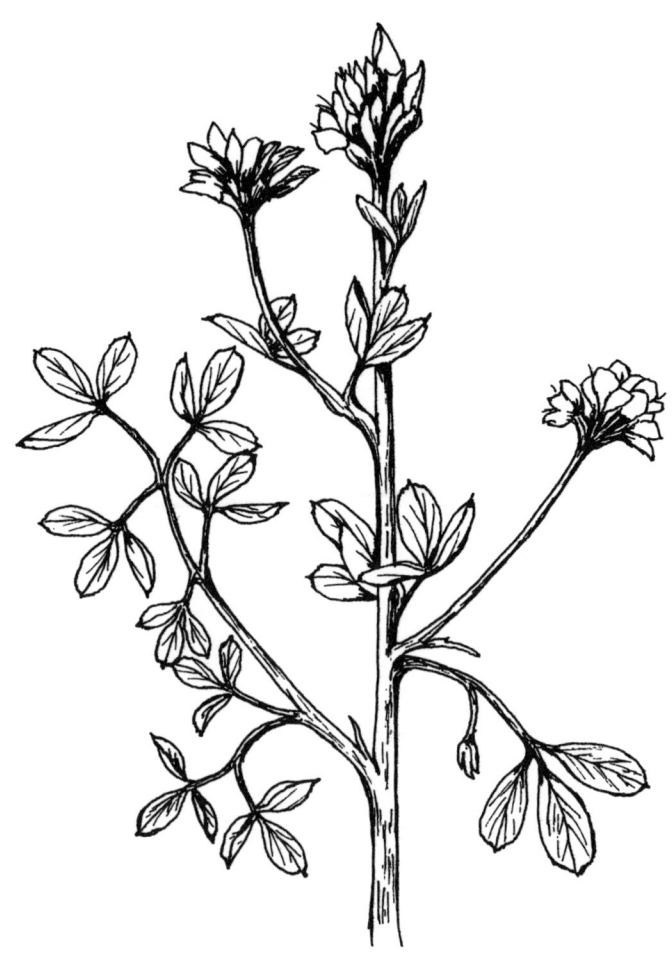

Alfalfa

The Herbs

Alfalfa (Medicago sativa)

Alfalfa relieves pain from inflammation and hay fever. It has been known to benefit the bladder and prostate. It is helpful in neutralizing uric acid of arthritis and bursitis. It is useful in eliminating cholesterol. The alkaloid in the leaves strengthens the central nervous system.

Aloe Vera (Aloe Vera)

The Aloe plant is known best for its ability to heal severe burns and irritated skin rashes. Aloe produces glowing skin when applied and helps to heal wounds by drawing out infection. It is effective in healing ulcers of the stomach and regulates the bowels. Aloe has been found by the Indians to have antibacterial abilities and has been used as an antibiotic.

Aloe Vera juice has been found to be beneficial in gastro-intestinal disorders including those of the stomach and colon.

Amaranth (Amaranthus hypochondriacus)

Amaranth is an astringent, meaning it is a contracting and drying herb. With these properties it is useful in diarrhea, dysentery, rectal bleeding and excessive menstruation. It can also be used for skin problems externally and for soothing of the mouth and throat.

Anise (Pimpinella anisum)

Anise has been known to improve appetite by stimulating the digestion. It increases the digestive juices and breaks down fat into fatty acids. Anise was first mentioned in Egyptian records dated 2,000 B.C. It is used to relieve wind from the large intestines and to promote milk in nursing mothers. Anise can be boiled in a half pint of milk and taken on a daily basis.

Arnica (Arnica montana)

Primarily used externally, Arnica is also used as a stimulant, diuretic, expectorant, emollient and vulnerary. Only a very small amount of Arnica need be used diluted because a tincture can cause inflammation and burn. It can be used as a poultice externally to relieve stomach cramps. Arnica is a favored ingredient in mouthwash when diluted and is excellent in the treatment of sore muscles and tendons.

Barberry (Berberis vulgaris)

Barberry is an excellent laxative and helps to increase bile production; therefore improving the function of the liver. The fresh juice of the Barberry strengthens the gums. The alkaloid in the root kills parasites and is an excellent anti-cancer herb. Barberry has also been used to benefit acne, arthritis and boils.

Barley (Hordeum vulgare)

Barley is a demulcent which means it soothes irritated tissues, particularly mucous membranes. Barley has been used successfully for stomach problems and intestinal blocks. It is excellent in the action on fevers and externally can be used for sores and tumors. Barley is good for those recovering from illness or weakness. It is high in Vitamins B and E. It is important in the treatment of asthma and bronchitis due to Hordenine, an alkaloid possessing properties like ephedrine produced in the root of the Barley plant.

Basil (Ocymum basilicum)

Basil is good for respiration problems due to nervousness and indigestion. Basil is the sacred plant of India and is said to open the heart and the mind. It is excellent in fighting colds and lung disorders. It removes mucus and increases absorption.

Bay (Laurus nobilis)

Dedicated by the Greeks to Apollo and Aesculapius, the god of medicine, the Bay Tree was said to be capable of bringing about health and happiness. The Bay Tree is considered the Tree of Protection and marks the entrance to many an herbal garden. Bay leaf is added to beans and soups as prevention from gas and indigestion. Used to relieve pain and swelling from arthritic joints, Oil of Bay is used in a poultice wrap. Bay Tree leaves heated in olive oil can produce this remedy.

Bayberry (Myrica cerifera)

Bayberry has been known to dispel colds and improve the voice. It opens the mind and the senses. It helps rid tumors in the female tract and is a strong germicidal which destroys bacteria. It is beneficial as a gargle for problems with bleeding gums. It can help with menstrual bleeding and has been used in cases of epilepsy.

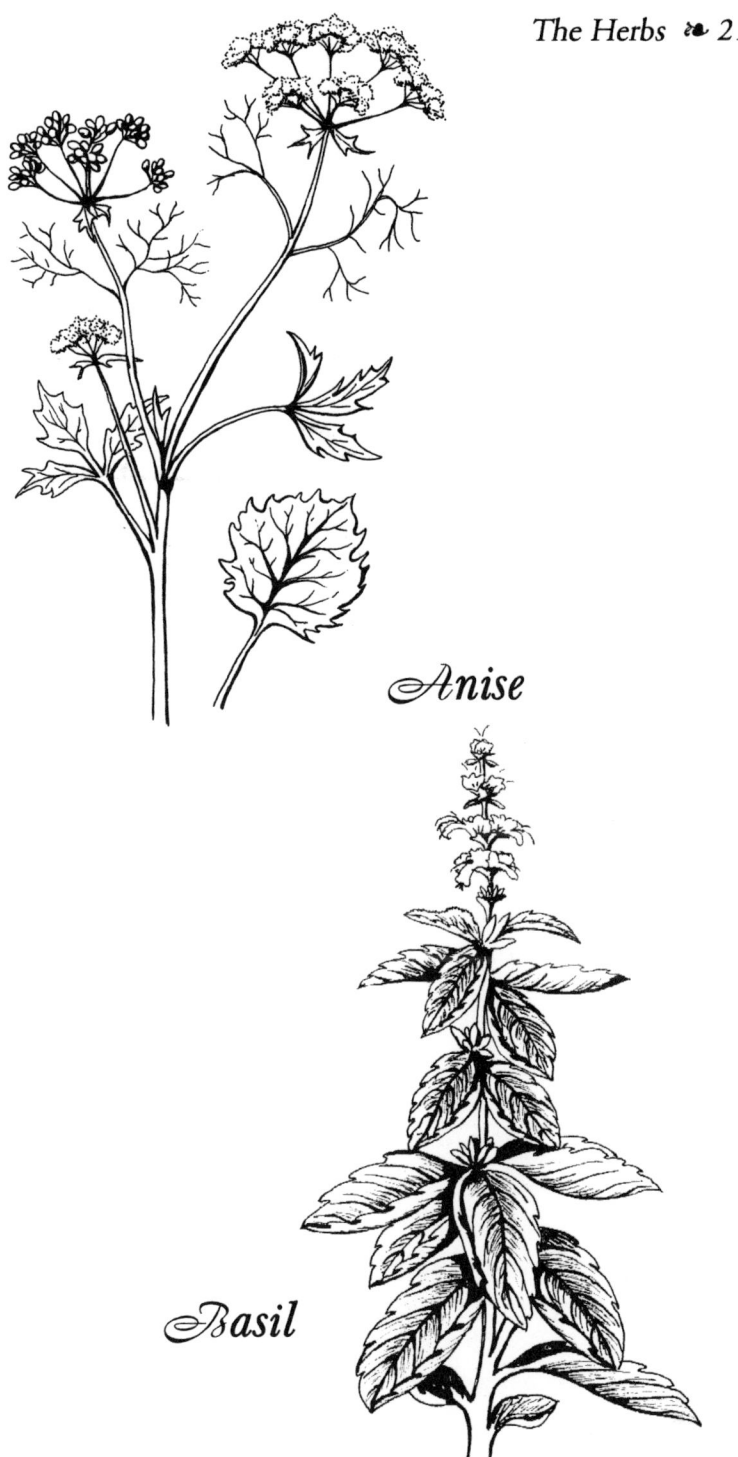

Anise

Basil

Bee Pollen

Bee Pollen is high in nutrients and has been shown by analysis to be able to sustain life. Hippocrates, the Father of Modern Medicine used Bee Pollen in his prescriptions to remedy a variety of maladies of the day. Greek Myth tells us that the sun and hornets married to create the bee, the ultimate nurturer. Bee Pollen has been shown to be an excellent anti-aging and energy supplement.

Black Cohosh (Cimicifuga racemosa)

Black Cohosh is used as a relaxing herb. It is considered an antispasmodic herb. Black Cohosh has been used to calm nervous tension in the muscles. Both the skeletal muscles and the smooth muscles of the internal organs are helped by Black Cohosh. It stimulates natural estrogen production and benefits women during menopause.

American Indians used Black Cohosh to treat women's complaints as well as rheumatism. Small doses can be used to treat children with diarrhea.

*WARNING: Large doses of Black Cohosh acts like poisoning.

Black Pepper (Piper nigrum)

Black pepper is a healing herb and according to the Indian Ayurvedic System, has properties of the sun. It is one of the most powerful digestive stimulants. It destroys waste build up. It will relieve congestion, headaches, and

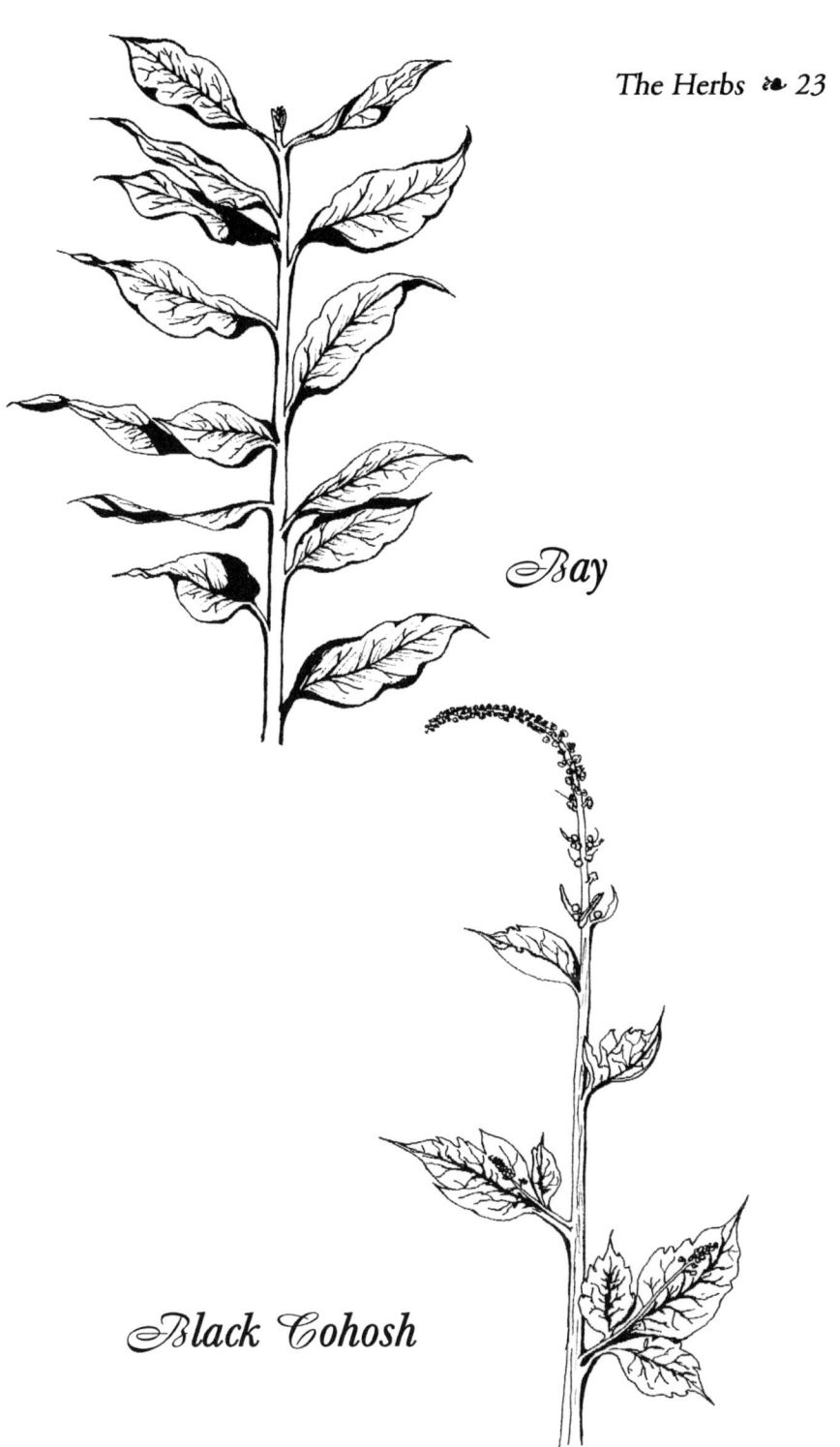

Bay

Black Cohosh

has even been known to relieve epileptic seizures by restoring oxygen to the brain. It is used to treat inflammation externally and will dry up secretions and rid the system of tumors. It has also been an excellent remedy for the first signs of disease, and has been used to help during menopause.

Blessed Thistle (Cnicus benedictus)

It is useful for relief of indigestion. It stimulates the heart, blood, mammary glands and the uterus. Blessed Thistle balances hormones and increases Mother's milk. It is good for menopause and any blockage of the menses. Blessed Thistle increases oxygen to the brain and helps circulation strengthening the memory and heart. It has been known to dispel tumors due to blockage. It stimulates the stomach and cleanses the liver.

Blue Cohosh (Caulophyllum thalictroides)

Blue Cohosh was used by the Native Americans to relieve menstrual cramps and pain and discomfort from childbirth. It was used to induce labor. Blue and Black Cohosh are sometimes combined and are beneficial in nervous conditions. Blue Cohosh and Black Cohosh act together as an antispasmodic on the entire system. Blue Cohosh is also a diuretic. These herbs are insoluble in water so they can be used in alcohol as a tincture in combination with each other. Blue Cohosh works on the

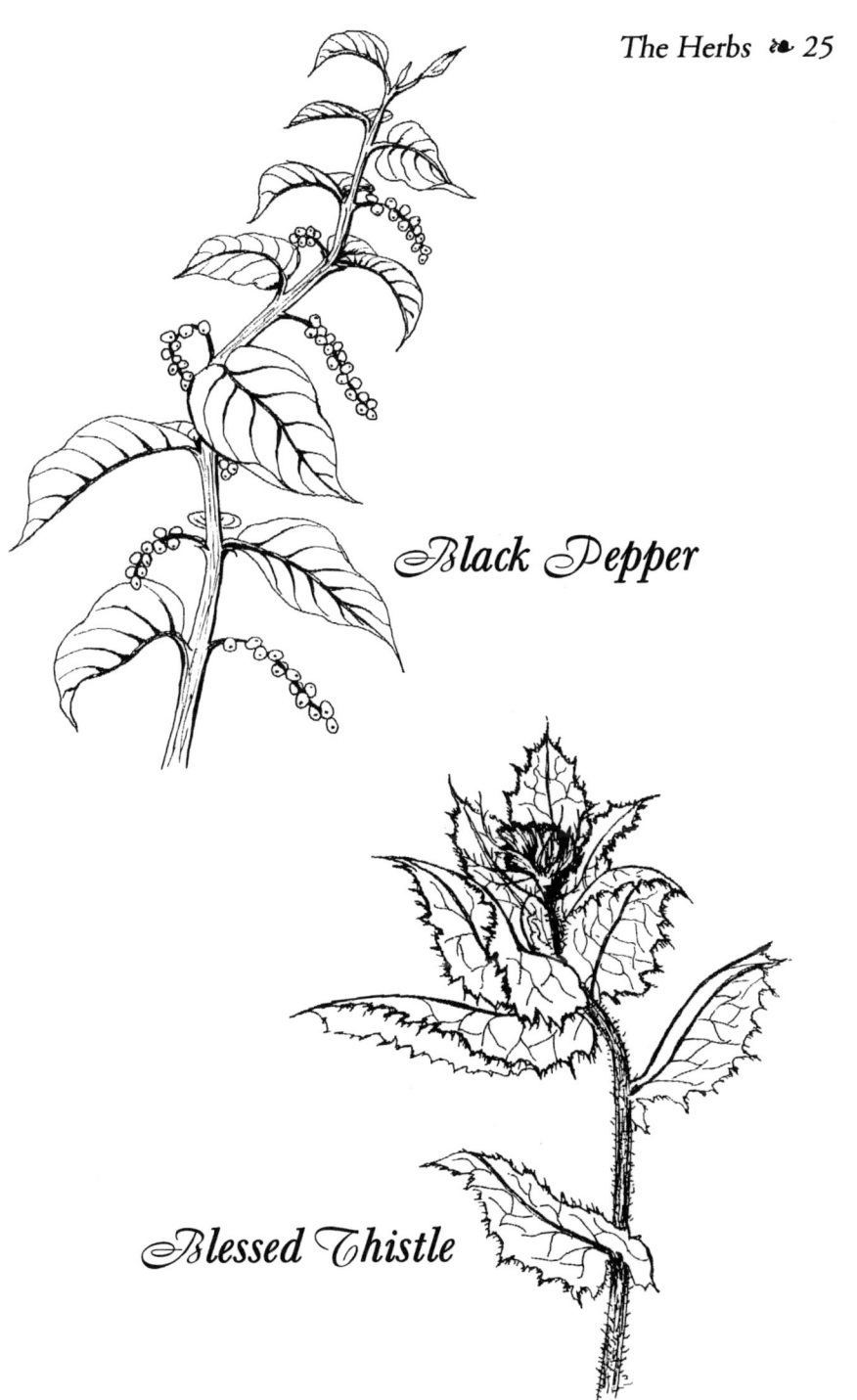

Black Pepper

Blessed Thistle

womb or uterus and the joints. Blue Cohosh is very irritating to the mucous membranes and can cause dermatitis.

*WARNING: Children have been poisoned by the berries. Use only under Medical advise.

Blue Flag (Iris versicolor)

Blue Flag stimulates the liver and can remove fluids in other areas of the body. It stimulates the heart which can purify the blood. Blue Flag is good for chronic vomiting, gastritis, liver and gallbladder and is good in removing blocks in sinuses. Historically used by the Indians for dropsy, Blue Flag is good at removing water from all over the body. It is good for migraines, especially when caused by stomach problems.

*WARNING: Because Blue Flag contains an acrid substance that acts on the gastro-intestinal tract, the liver and the pancreas, it can cause rashes.

Blue Vervain (Verbena hastata)

Blue Vervain is a natural sedative and has properties that aid in nervous disorders. Taken as a tea it will fight fevers and colds and is particularly helpful in conditions of congestion in the chest and the throat. It historically has been named Indian Hyssop, Traveler's Joy and Wild Hyssop.

Blue Flag

Blue Vervain

Boneset (Eupatorium perfoliatum)

Boneset is used to treat colds and fever and its name is derived from the effect it has in aiding bones to heal. Taken hot it has the effect of breaking up congestion and chill, while cold gives the infusion a laxative property.

Borage (Borago officinalis)

Borage is an excellent and gentle diuretic. It is good for reducing swelling. Borage historically was known to be an herb for the heart and is excellent to lift the spirits and make the heart happy through strengthening. It is taken as a tea for lung problems. Borage is used for all irritations of the skin and mucous membranes. From May to September, the Celts used Borage with wine to increase production of adrenalin in the blood. In modern preparations Borage is used to reduce nervous tension. It can be used as a tincture or as an ingredient in a salve.

Burdock (Arctium lappa)

Burdock is an excellent blood purifier. It is helpful to the kidneys in promoting filtering of impurities. Burdock is historically used to neutralize poisons. For liver problems, the leaves will best stimulate the secretion of bile. The fresh leaves can be used as a remedy for poison ivy or oak. It has been proven to treat boils, acne and eczema with great success.

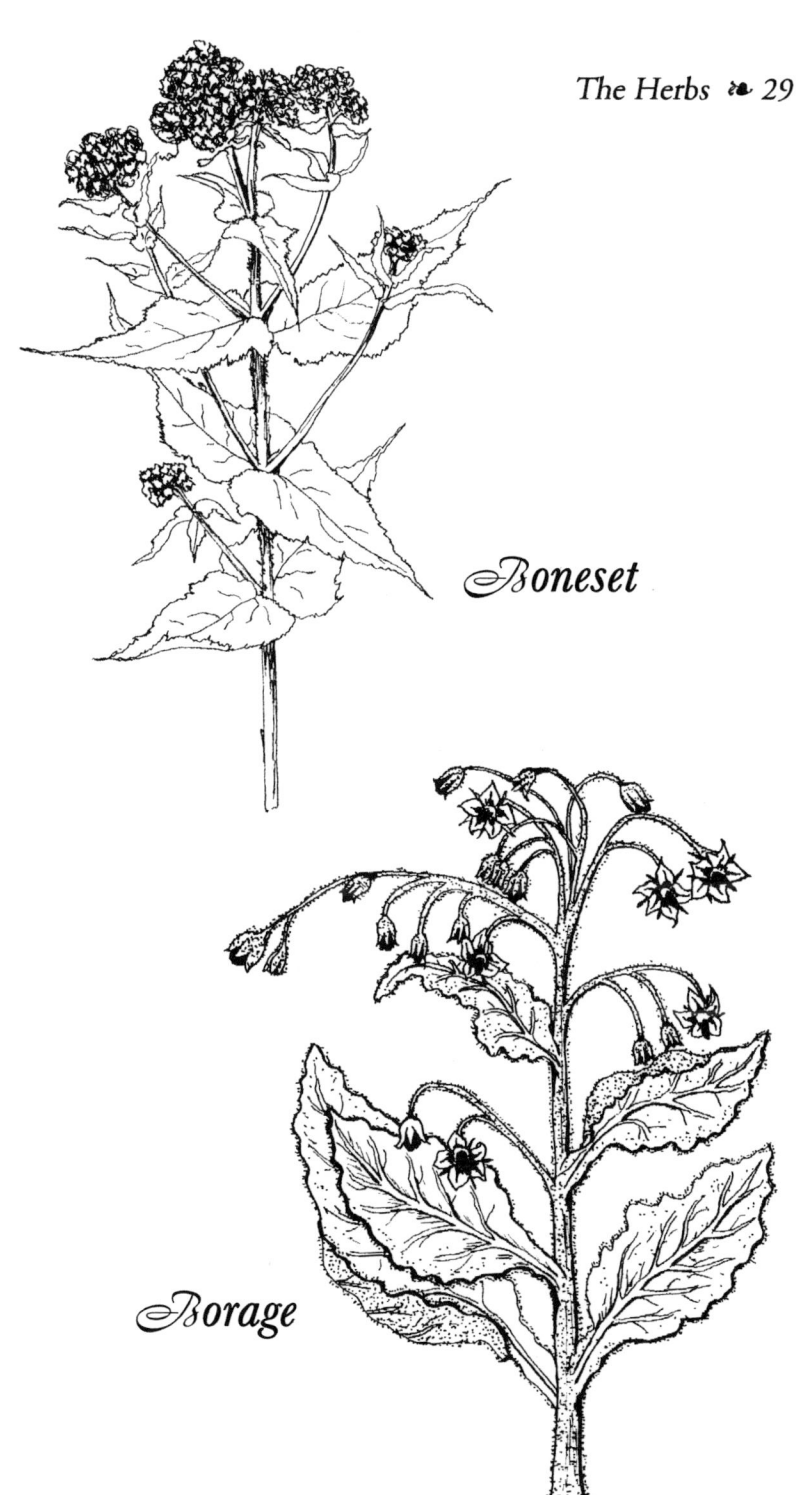

Boneset

Borage

Calendula/Marigold (Calendula officinalis)

Calendula is beneficial to the blood and the skin. It has been used historically in cases of smallpox, measles, bee stings and other eruptive skin diseases. Calendula can be taken internally for fevers, boils and to prevent vomiting. It relieves inflammation externally.

Caraway Seeds (Carum carvi)

The roots of the Caraway Seed plant can strengthen the stomach. The root can be applied with pulverized seeds as a hot compress to the stomach to ease indigestion pain. Historically Caraway Seeds have helped children with digestive problems. They increase urine and are said to sharpen eyesight.

Cardamom (Elettaria cardamomum)

Cardamom is one of the best digestive stimulants. It removes water and mucus from the stomach and lungs. It stimulates the mind and the heart. Cardamom added to milk will neutralize mucus-forming properties of the milk and detoxify coffee. It is good for the nerves and over acidity.

Castor Bean (Ricinus communis)

The oil pressed from the Castor Bean is the most widely

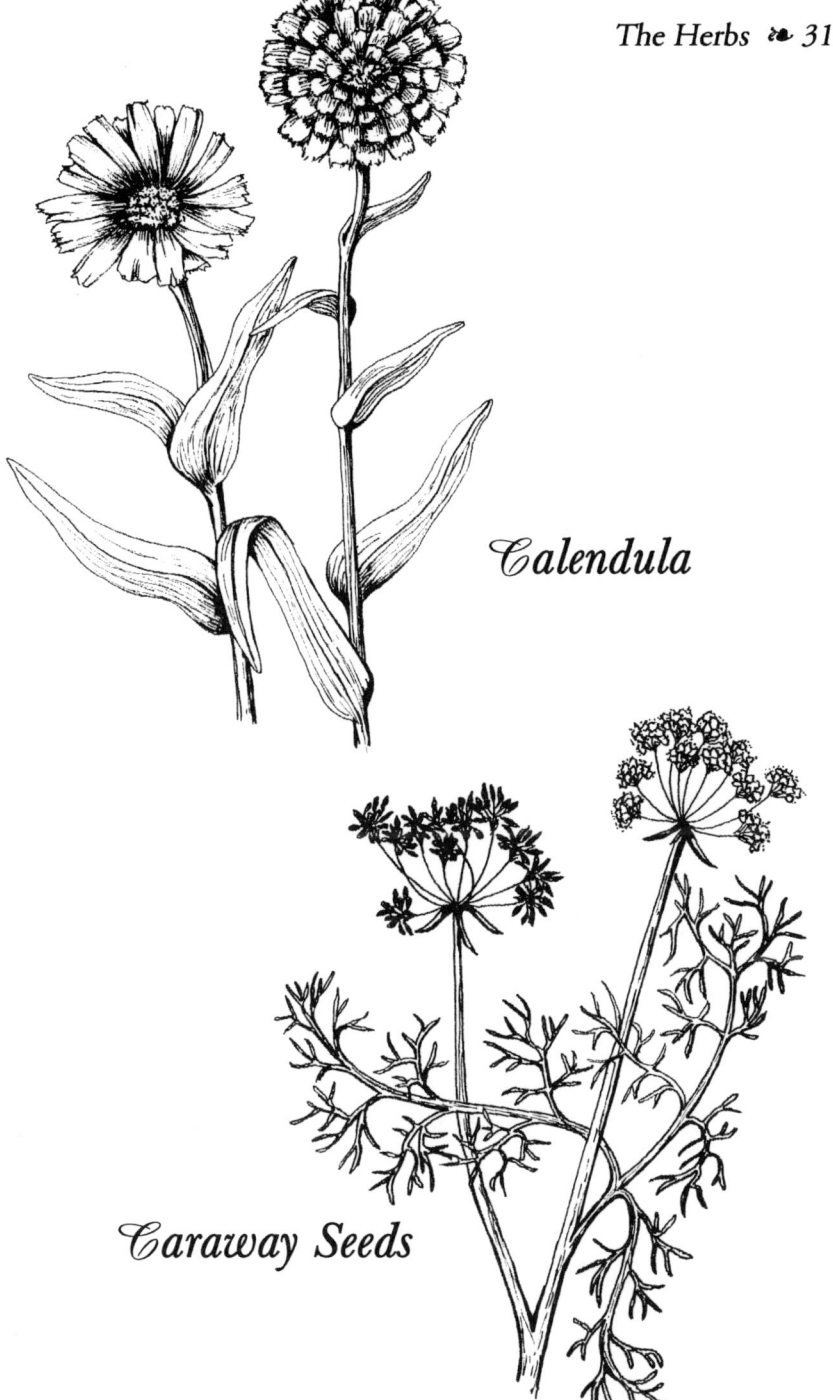

Calendula

Caraway Seeds

known purgative--Castor Oil. The oil is the only part of the plant that should be used, in that the entire plant and seed contains a poison to the blood. When extracting the oil the poison remains in the seed.

Catnip (Nepeta cataria)

It is used for nerves and the intestines. It is a mild antispasmodic herb. Catnip is an excellent teething tea for children. It has a calming effect on stomach cramps, spasms, gas, hiccoughs and any nervous disorders.

Catnip has been used historically as a mild tranquilizer and has been used successfully to fight insomnia.

Cayenne/Capsicum (Capsicum fontescens)

Cayenne is of benefit to the heart and circulation. It is used as a crisis herb to stop bleeding and heart attacks. Strokes and any condition of low vitality are aided by the increased circulation that Cayenne brings about. Depression and arthritis are both helped by the increased circulation that Cayenne Pepper brings about.

Celandine (Chelidonium majus) The Greater

It purifies the blood and is an excellent application for corns and warts. It can also be used as an eye lotion. Historically, Celandine was used as a rub with Chamomile to take away griping pains in the stomach and pains associated

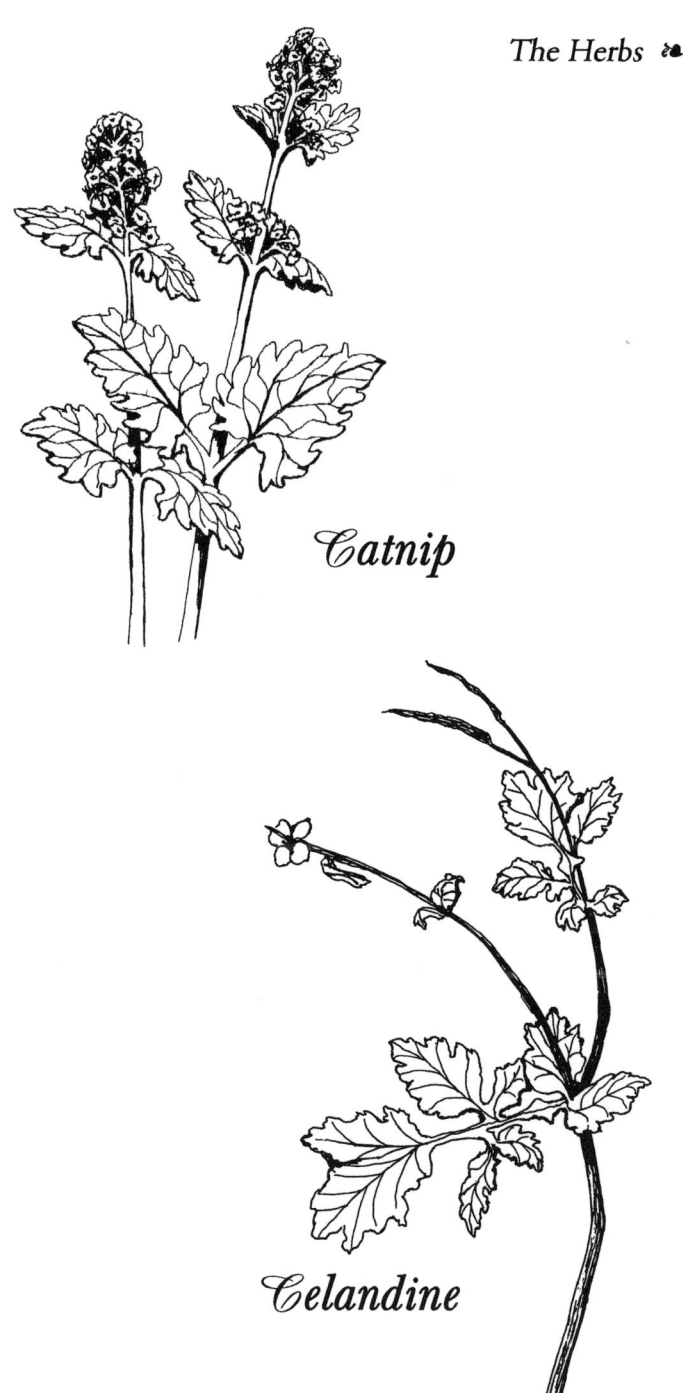

Catnip

Celandine

with pregnancy. Also, Celandine was used to help with menstrual pain, and was applied to women's breasts to stop menses. Celandine has a good effect on digestive, stomach, gall bladder and liver problems. It can treat skin disease like herpes, eczema and ring worm.

*CAUTION: The juice is very dangerous and has produced skin poisoning from touching the plant. Also, it can be poison to the lungs and liver producing congestion. It has a narcotic effect on the nervous system.

Chamomile (Anthemis nobilis)

Nerves, stomach, kidneys, liver, uterus and circulation are all benefited by Chamomile. Chamomile has tryptophan in it and has been used for its soothing effect to counteract insomnia and quiet the stomach or nerves. Tryptophan is an amino acid that regulates sleep and mood patterns. It is particularly beneficial to treat digestive disorders. Chamomile acts as an anti-inflammatory which helps to relax agitation in children or adults. It makes a good wash for wounds that are slow in healing or for stiff and painful joints.

Chervil (Myrrhis odorata)

Chervil is used to warm the stomach and expel wind from the stomach. It can be used as an expectorant and, therefore, is good in treating a cough. Historically Chervil was used to treat the plague because its roots are antiseptic. The juice was said to heal ulcers of the head and face.

Chickweed (Stellaria media)

Chickweed is a soothing agent that can be made into a poultice to relieve swelling and bronchial conditions. It is a cooling herb and can be used to treat inflamed skin or tissues that result in skin diseases. Chickweed is good for hemorrhoids, excema, ulcers or psoriasis.

Chicory (Cichorium intybus)

Chicory is used as an appetizer to stimulate digestive juices. It is historically used to fight jaundice and for spleen problems. The glands respond well to Chicory in the digestive organs. Also used to treat inflammation, Chicory flowers and leaves can be applied in a wrapped cloth to the afflicted area.

Chives (Allium schoenoprasum)

Chives are rich in sulphur and can increase or start urine to flow. Chives are considered to be antibiotic. They stimulate the appetite and have been known to have a good action on the kidneys as well as strengthening the stomach.

Cinnamon (Cinnamonium zeylanicum)

Cinnamon is stimulating and warms the system. It is useful to balance cooling foods such as fruits, milk and desserts. Cinnamon is known to warm the organs and to treat diarrhea, cramps, the heart and abdominal pains. Cinnamon is excellent for coughs, wheezing and low back pains.

Coffee Berry (Rhamnus californica)

The Coffee Berry is especially useful for inflammatory conditions of rheumatism when joints become swollen and painful. It is a mild stimulant used for the liver and can increase bile production.

Comfrey (Symphytum officinale)

Comfrey is used for ulcers and colitis. It has been used both internally and externally for healing of bone breaks, unhealed wounds and internal ulcers. Comfrey treats the bones, skin, muscles, and cleans up dead tissues. Because it is a demulcent it is used to benefit the lungs. It suppresses bleeding and heals the respiratory system. Comfrey helps the pancreas to regulate blood sugar levels.

Coriander/Cilantro (Coriandrum sativum)

Coriander has been used as an appetizer, aromatic and as an antispasmodic. It relieves rheumatism and painful joints through external application of a poultice. Historically, Coriander was considered an aphrodisiac.

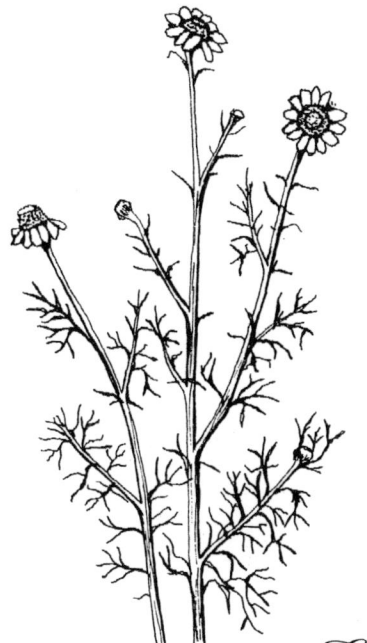

Chamomile

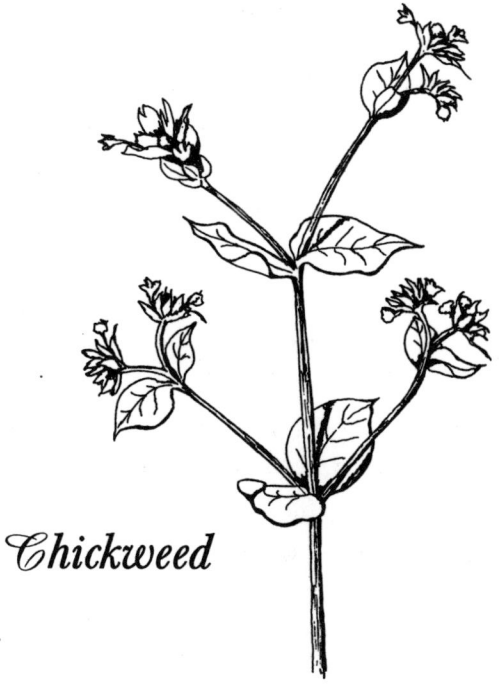

Chickweed

Cornsilk (Stigmata maidis)

Cornsilk contains large amounts of Vitamin K, known to be a clotting agent that helps to control bleeding. It is also beneficial in cleaning the urinary tract.

Cucumber (Cucumis sativus)

The juice of the Cucumber can be used as a beauty aid for skin and eyes. It is an excellent diuretic and is important and beneficial to the kidneys and rheumatic conditions. Cucumber has been used successfully and with great benefit to help the intestines, lungs, kidneys and skin.

Cumin (Cuminum cyminum)

Cumin acts as a stimulant and as an antispasmodic. The seeds can be used to increase breast milk. It has been successfully used as a liniment for stimulating circulation. Cumin is used to aid in indigestion and is a main ingredient in curry.

Cyclamen (Cyclamen europaeum)

This is a very excessive purgative and was used historically in Europe for dropsy and mucous congestions. Cyclamen has been known to heal wounds that are purulent and to fight intestinal worms.

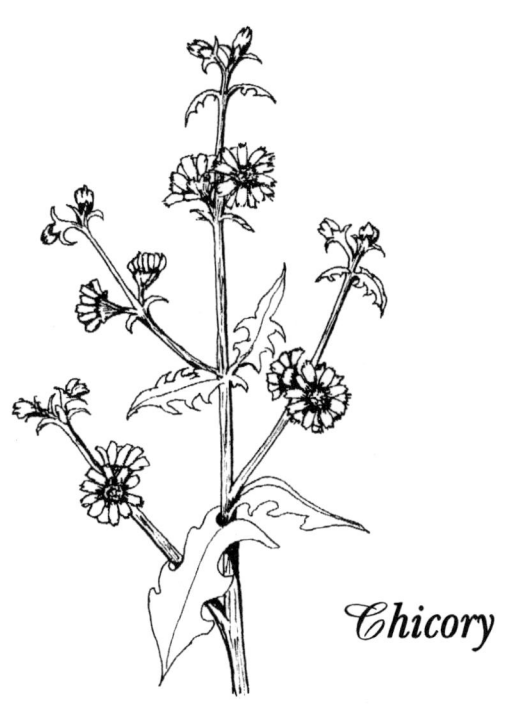

Chicory

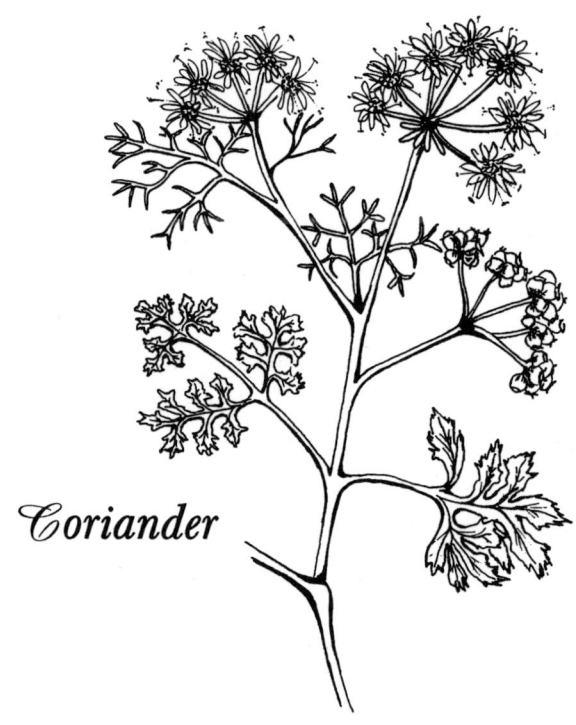

Coriander

*CAUTION: Cyclamen is poisonous and was used to coat arrowheads for poisonous spears.

Damiana (Turnera aphrodisiaca)

Damiana is used for the reproductive organs, nerves and kidneys. It has been known to stimulate the male hormone, testosterone. Small amounts of Damiana can act as a tonic to the nervous system. Damiana is of benefit in depression, low energy, impotence and nervous conditions. Parkinson's Disease and Prostate problems have been aided by Damiana. It acts as a brain tonic. It acts as an overall tonic to the entire nervous system.

Dandelion (Taraxacum officinale)

Dandelion stimulates the liver, kidneys, gall bladder, stomach, pancreas, and intestines. For the blood, Dandelion is considered a nutritive herb. It is known as a Spring Tonic due to its rich source of vitamins and minerals. Dandelion is soothing to the digestive tract and promotes healing. It absorbs toxins, removes water and increases bile production. Dandelion has been historically helpful with gout and rheumatism. Because of its stimulating and soothing qualities it has been used to great benefit on swollen joints, and in cases of jaundice and any problems involving the liver.

It works on tumors and cysts in the breasts particularly when these problems are related to suppression of lactation. It helps sores that do not heal, hepatitis, diabetes and edema. It is a good blood purifier and heals inflammation.

Dill (Anethum graveolens)

Dill dispels wind from the stomach and is excellent for digestive upsets, particularly the Oil-of-Dill. Historically the seeds have been used for flavoring food and the plant can be used on foods to make them less difficult to digest. To help stimulate the appetite and to stimulate the flow for nursing mothers, Dill has an excellent effect. It also helps to eliminate bad breath by chewing the seeds.

Dong Quai (Angelica sinensis)

This herb has been used for centuries by the Chinese to help in menopause. It is of benefit to the uterus, blood, muscles, nerves and has been used for all female problems. Migraine headaches, liver problems and heart palpitations are all benefited by Dong Quai. It has been known to dissolve blood clots and to nourish the brain and strengthen the entire central nervous system. It has been known to help in insomnia and hypertension. Because it is an antispasmodic it helps relieve cramps. It should not be used during heavy menstrual flow or in pregnancy.

Echinacea (Echinacea angustifolia)

Echinacea is known as a Blood Purifier and can be

used for skin conditions such as eczema, acne or boils. It can also be used for promoting digestion. It is an enhancer for the immune system and acts on the kidneys and lymph glands. It fights viral infestations and bacteria and is good for upper respiratory infections, tonsillitis, laryngitis, and sinus infections. It is also a good mouth rinse for pyorrhea and gingivitis.

Ephedra (Ephedra sinica)

Ephedra is also Ma Huang and has been known as a remedy for kidney and bladder problems since early pioneers first used it as a blood purifier. Native Americans used it to treat syphilis. It has been used to benefit asthma, bronchitis, and other conditions of constriction or congestion. It is a strong stimulant and increases the function of the adrenals. Ephedra should only be used in conditions where the individual is strong and not weak from illness. Because it acts on the body like adrenaline, it is a powerful mucus reducing herb and promotes alertness and wakefulness.

Evening Primrose (Oenothera biennis)

Evening Primrose is an astringent and a mucilaginous. This means that it causes tissue to contract and dry up, but it also has a gelatinous consistency. It is important for women in menopause and helps mental depression. It stimulates the liver, spleen, and digestion. Externally it can be used in a salve for rashes and other skin irritations.

Eyebright (Euphrasia officinalis)

Eyes, blood and liver are all benefited by Eyebright. It is a cooling herb and detoxifies. It has been known to stimulate the liver which clears up the eyes and vision. It is cooling and removes heat. It is also beneficial in cases where there is inflammation of the nose and throat.

Fennel (Foeniculum vulgare)

Both the seed and the root can be used to benefit the stomach function to relieve cramping and to expel gas. It removes waste materials and strengthens the nerves. Fennel has been used to increase the appetite. It has been of benefit to nursing mothers to stimulate milk and to purify the blood.

Flax (Linum usitatissimum)

The seed strengthens the healing of the lung tissue and promotes healing. The seeds are known as linseeds. Specifically good for the lungs and lung diseases, such as asthma and consumption it also helps colic. Historically Flax seeds were found in Egyptian tombs. The seeds are soothing and can be used as a laxative. An infusion of Flax seeds can be used for inflammatory bowel, such as colitis and inflammation of urinary tract or skin externally.

Foxglove (Digitalis purpurea)

It is used to regulate and stimulate cardiac activity. Digitalis is deadly poisonous if taken to excess.

Garlic (Allium sativum)

Garlic is of benefit to the respiratory system, the circulation and the digestion. It is helpful to the nerves and the sinuses and kills infection. Garlic acts against bacteria and parasites and builds intestinal flora. It has been shown by modern studies to build the immune system and to play a major role in fighting heart disease. Garlic has proven to be helpful to fight candida yeast infections and to normalize blood pressure. It can relax the heart muscle and release blocks.

Ginger (Zingiber officinale)

Ginger stimulates the stomach, intestines and joints. It improves the circulation and digestion. It can strengthen the circulation externally and can be used in a poultice to help remove inflammation from arthritic joints. It is one of the most widely used stimulants and promotes cleansing through perspiration. It is useful to start suppressed menstruation. It can be used to counteract seasickness or diarrhea and has been known to stop flu symptoms. Ginger combined with Bayberry can protect against viruses. As an external poultice, Ginger can stimulate circulation in joints and relieve pain and swelling.

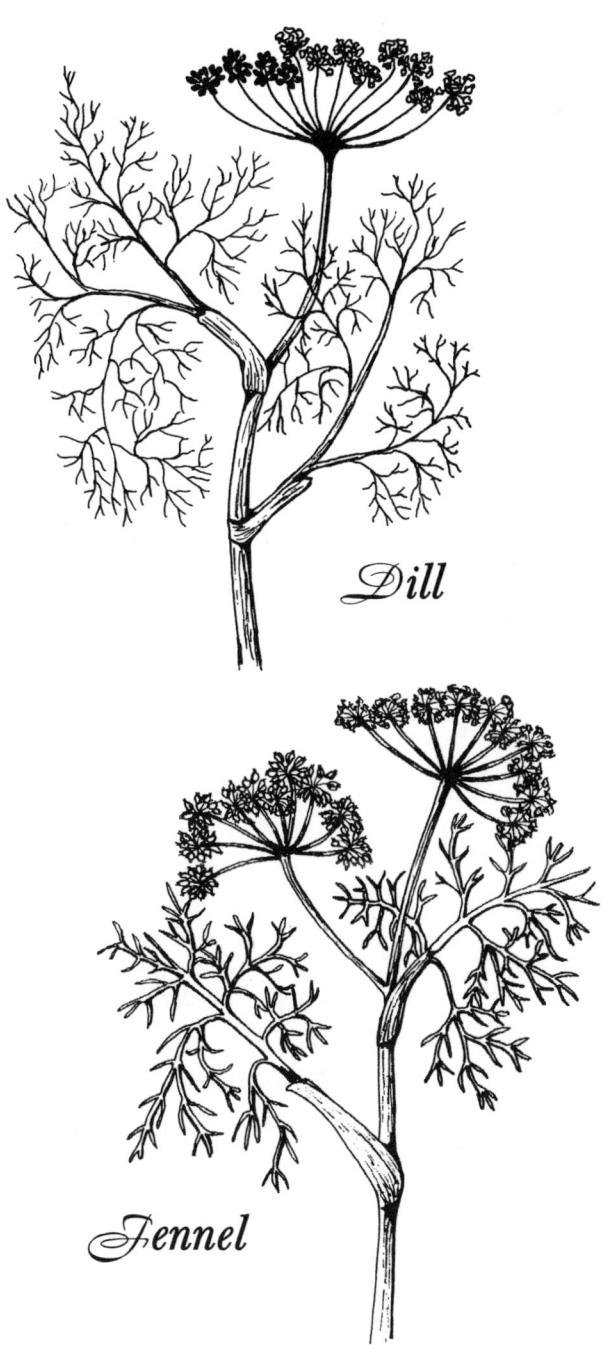

Dill

Fennel

Ginseng (Panax jen-sheng)

From the Chinese, this herb is a strong tonic to aid in heart action and body circulation. It has been known to increase accuracy in work involving the brain due to increased circulation. It benefits the whole body. It will normalize blood pressure but should not be used where there is inflammation or fever. It is useful to combat stress and increase concentration and physical efficiency. Native American tribes have been known to use American Ginseng in love potions. The American Ginseng has a milder effect. Ginseng has been known to reduce blood sugar levels and is good for diabetes. Ginseng should not be used if there is an excessive menstrual flow.

Golden Seal (Hydrastis canadensis)

Golden Seal has historically been used as a de-toxifyer aiding in stopping cold and flu symptoms through releasing toxins. Used as a gargle for sore throat and as a mouthwash for pyorrhea, Golden Seal has been known to heal mouth sores and sore gums.

It can be used as a laxative and acts directly on mucous membranes. Ringworm, bruises, wounds all respond to Golden Seal. Golden Seal has been known to stop bleeding and can be used as an external skinwash for erysipelas. After using tea as a wash, use powdered root of Golden Seal on sores.

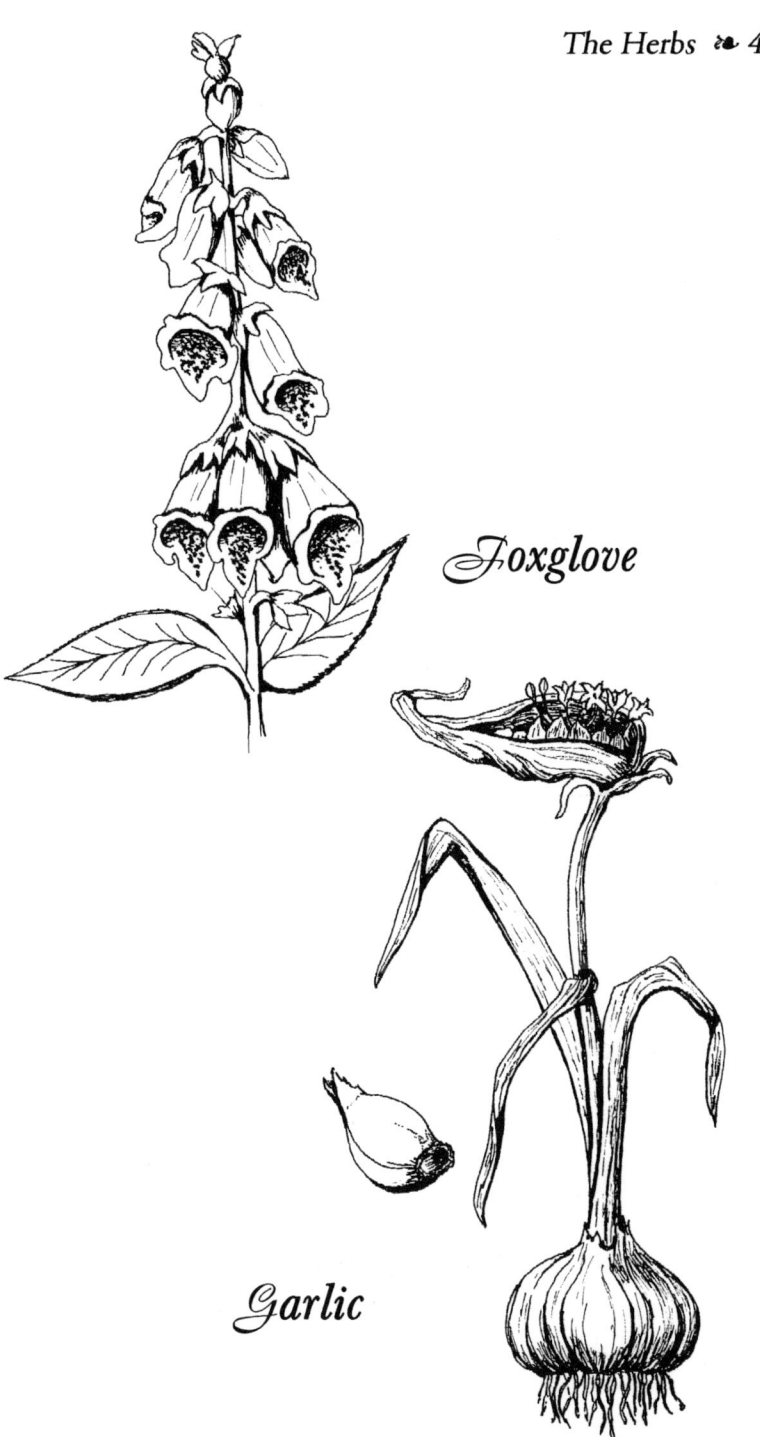

Foxglove

Garlic

Gotu Kola (Hydrocotyle asiatica)

Gotu Kola is used to strengthen the heart as well as the brain and memory. It has been known to balance hormones and improve stamina. Gotu Kola increases energy reserves and is beneficial to help relieve stress. Gotu Kola is the most widely used herb in the Ayurvedic System of India. It is called "Brahmi" by the East Indians and is considered to be the best nerve tonic. Its action is mainly towards the mind and the nerve disorders including schizophrenia and epilepsy. To the East Indian, Gotu Kola is used to increase longevity based on records dated thousands of years ago. It is said to neutralize acids of the blood and is considered beneficial to the kidneys, bladder, heart and increases circulation.

Hops (Humulus americanus)

Hops is a sedative and acts as an antibiotic as well. It has a good action on a nervous stomach. Hops has been known to relieve insomnia and indigestion. Externally, hops can be used on staph and other bacteria with a good action. As part of the beer-making process, hops is used as a preservative.

Horseradish (Armoracia lapathifolia)

Horseradish is a diuretic, a rubefacient and a stomachic. Because it is a diuretic it has a good action on rheumatic problems with removing excess water. Also, bladder constrictions and lower digestive problems in the colon and intestines are greatly benefited by Horseradish.

Hyssop (Hyssopus officinalis)

Hyssop is used mainly in lung conditions to expel mucus. It can be used as a stimulant to increase circulation. Hyssop can be used like Sage. It is helpful in diseases of inflammation and can be used to help burns and other skin problems. It historically has been used in cases of jaundice and dropsy. For treatment of poor digestion, make a tea.

Irish Moss (Chondrus crispus)

Irish Moss works on the respiratory and urinary systems. Seaweeds in general are important for deficiency. Irish Moss soothes inflamed membranes due to feeble conditions. Thyroid deficiencies are benefited with Irish Moss as it increases body fluids and enriches the body with minerals.

Jasmine (Jasminum officinale)

The old Herbals say the flower of the Jasmine can be used to calm the nerves. In the Orient, Jasmine was considered an aphrodisiac. In India, it is known as a cure for snakebite. It can be usually drunk in a tea and its gentle, cooling, sweetening properties are calming to the body. It is a subtle herb and a very potent one. Its strength acts as an anti-bacterial, anti-viral and anti-tumor agent. Especially important for women, Jasmine is considered a Yin herb and its flower is used to strengthen the lymphatic system.

Juniper (Juniperus communis)

Juniper is an antiseptic, carminative, diuretic and stomachic and a tonic. Juniper Berries are good for eliminating excess water and therefore good for gout and rheumatism.

Juniper Berries can be used to aid indigestion and to act on gastro-intestinal infections. Juniper Oil penetrates the skin easily and can be good for joint swellings by applying oil in a poultice to the effected area. Historically the berries of the Juniper have been used for "pains in the belly, coughs, shortness of breath..." and have been known to be of good benefit to women recovering from child-birth.

Khus-Khus (Vetiveria zizanioides)

Commonly known as Vetiver, this plant is used as an aromatic and made into perfume. It is also a stimulant and a tonic. Mostly used as a cosmetic or aromatic, the Vetiver has important use historically as a tonic when made into a tea.

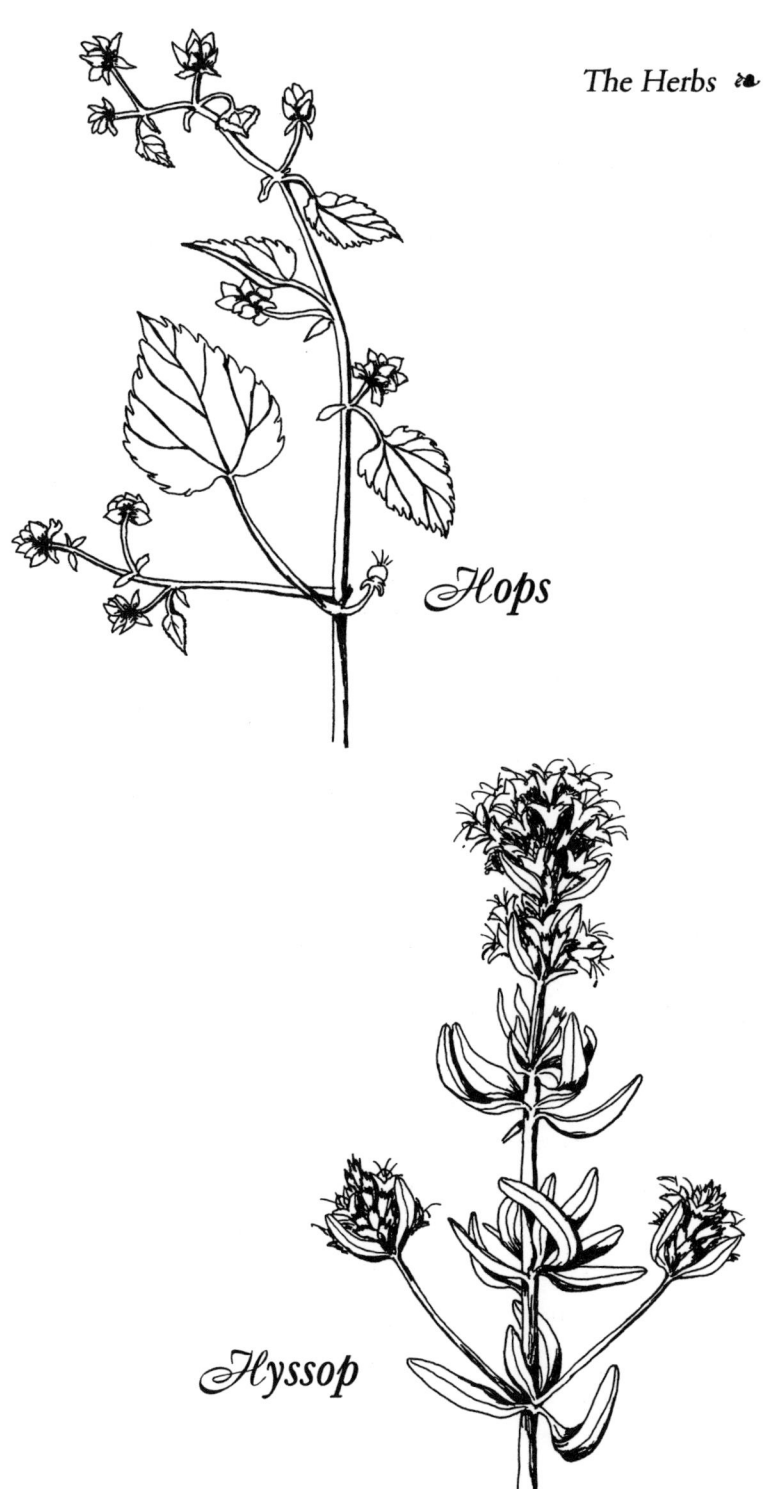

Hops

Hyssop

Kola Tree (Cola acuminata)

This is a tree that has become commonly known in our modern society as a stimulant among "soft drink" users. The tree grows in Africa and is cultivated in South America and the West Indies. It is used as a stimulant and a tonic. Containing more caffeine than the coffee berry, Kola nuts are used to combat fatigue and increase circulation to the brain and consequently eliminate headaches.

Lady's Slipper (Cypripedium pubescens)

Lady's Slipper helps with nervous headaches and irritability. It is of great benefit in chronic nervous conditions such as stroke. Lady's Slipper can be used to aid healing of the nerve sheath. It has been used in liver problems in combination with dandelion.

Lavender (Lavandula angustifolia)

Lavender was used in history as a cure for cramps, convulsions, faintings and to cure the restlessness of children. Distilled water with the flowers of Lavender was said to help a lost voice return.

Lavender is a stimulant and carminative. It has aromatic properties and is largely used in modern lotions and creams. Lavender will reduce nervousness when used as an oil in baths and can be placed on the pillow as a cure for insomnia. For fussing children place in a bag underneath the pillow to relax and promote quiet. Lavender has a

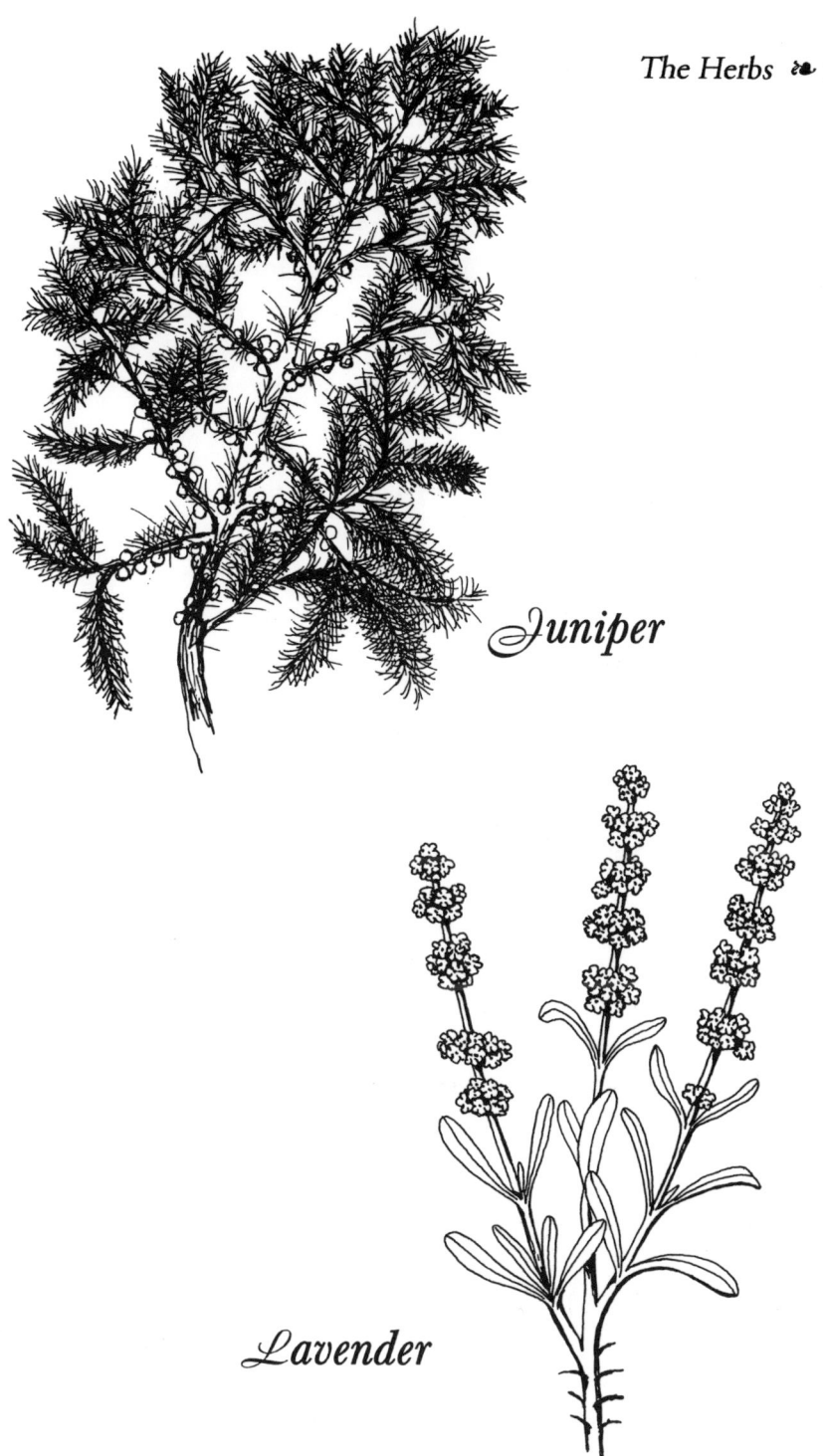

Juniper

Lavender

direct and relaxing effect on the heart and so has been used successfully to lower blood pressure. It is good for skin diseases as an ingredient in oils, and has been known to help in rheumatic conditions. Used as an oil for massage therapy, the relaxing effect on the heart helps relax the muscles as well. Historically, Lavender was used for "palsies."

Lemon Balm (Melissa officinalis)

Lemon Balm is a cooling herb. It is used to aid with the nerves and with circulation. Historically Lemon Balm has been used to fight melancholy and to promote acceptance. It has been used with children to great success and is considered a good herb to ward off fever.

Lettuce (Lactuca sativa)

Lettuce, historically, has been used as an oil to help sleep. Even in its plant form it provides a cooling, soothing effect that acts on the blood in such a way that sleep is promoted. It has been used in an application to the region of the heart and liver to reduce heat. Many English Homeopaths believe that lettuce can help cure impotence.

Licorice (Glycyrrhiza glabra)

Licorice is a wonderful herb to help the body cope with stress. It can be used for peptic ulcers. It relaxes the organs so the body can produce estrogen and acts as an emulsifier. It nourishes the adrenals. It can be used for sore throat and hoarseness. It has been used primarily for bronchial problems. It has a good action on the lungs, spleen, and liver.

Lily (Garden) (Lilium candidum)

Historically this Lily was used to fight fevers and the dropsy. For scalds and burns it was used in a salve. It was used for women who had difficulty in childbirth and particularly to dispel the afterbirth. It is an astringent, meaning it drys up and contracts tissue and can be used externally for ulcers and vaginal discharge.

Lily (Water) (Nymphaea alba)

Lily is a strong astringent and will stop diarrhea. It has been used successfully in inflammatory conditions, boils, ulcers combined with Slippery Elm. Historically, the Lily was used to take away freckles and sunburn. It can stop leucorrhea if used in the vagina.

Lobelia (Lobelia inflata)

History shows Lobelia to be used in connection with whooping cough and asthma. It is good for spasmodic lungs and respiratory conditions. It can bring about vomiting. Its action is on the nerves, lungs, stomach, muscles, circulation and can be used for a dry cough. Lobelia can be rubbed on gums of teething children. It loosens hard mucus and can be used in small doses effectively.

*CAUTION: Small doses of Lobelia is considered most effective in that it is toxic and can cause overdose.

Lovage (Levisticum officinale)

Lovage has been used to increase elimination. It can ease painful menstruation. The root has been used to expel wind from the stomach. It should not be used by pregnant women because it can bring on the menses.

*CAUTION: In heavy doses Lovage can cause kidney damage.

Magnolia (Magnolia glauca)

Magnolia has been known to be good for skin diseases. Historically, it was said that Magnolia helped people quit smoking tobacco. Magnolia can be made into a tea by using the bark and steeping in boiled water.

Maidenhair (Adiantum pedatum)

The Maidenhair fern is used as a tonic and has been known to be used to break up congestion and other colds and flus. Used as a hair rinse, it will act as a tonic to the scalp and subsequently increase hair growth. It can be used for asthma, bronchitis, pleurisy, and acts as a gentle

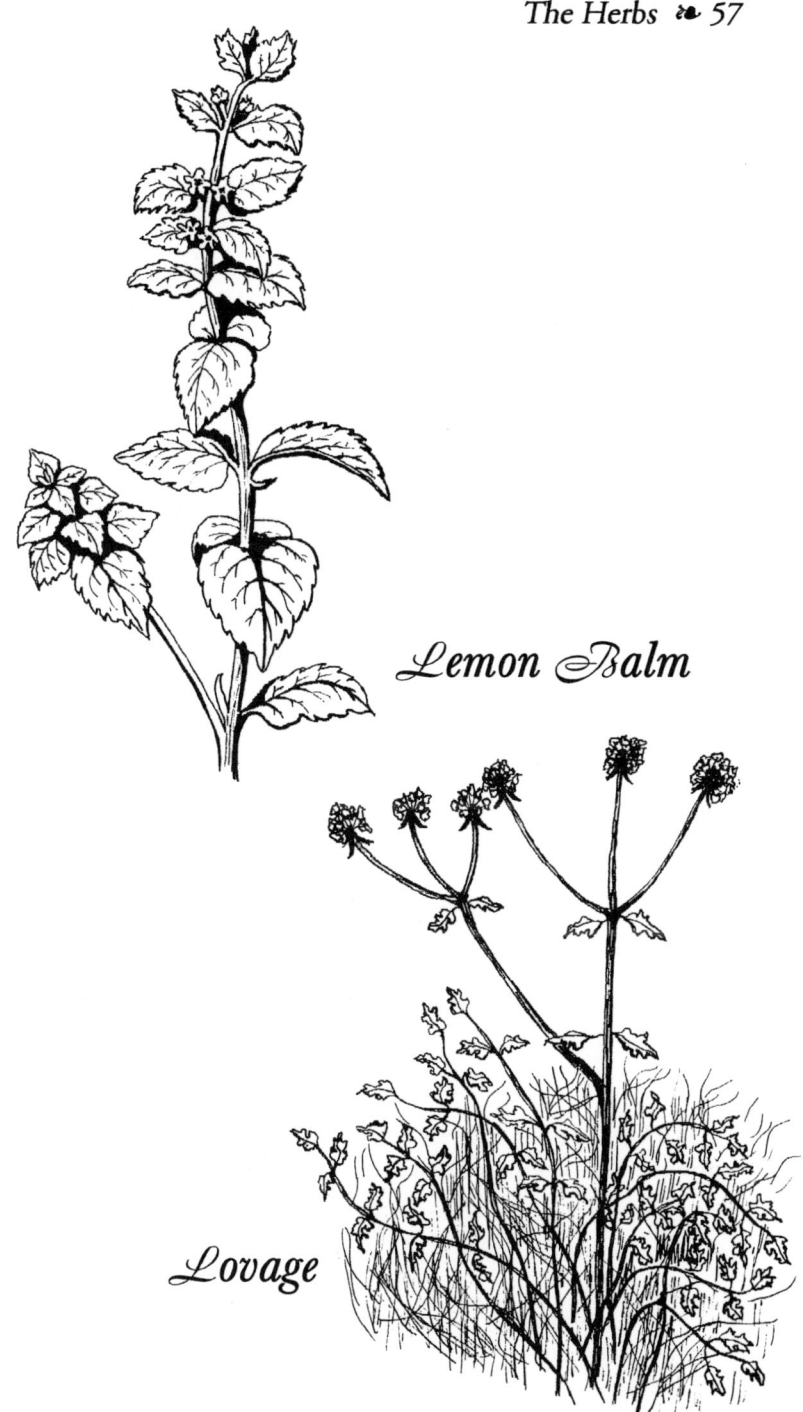

Lemon Balm

Lovage

diuretic which benefits the kidneys.

Mandrake (Podohyllum peltatum)

This reference is to the American Mandrake in contrast to the European variety which has no relation. The Native Americans used the root of the Mandrake to break up hard mucus. It is a very strong purgative. Known for its fruit, which is poisonous, Native Americans sometimes used the Mandrake to kill themselves. The Mandrake's leaves are cooling, however, and medicinally have been used for ointments to treat skin conditions.

*WARNING: The root should not be used for domestic use. Use only under professional advisement.

Marjoram (Marjorana hortensis)

For diseases that cause coldness in the head or stomach, or chest, Sweet Marjoram can warm and comfort the afflicted area. Also, Sweet Marjoram has been known to be good for gastritis, and the use of an oil can be rubbed on stiff joints. Sweet Marjoram has been known to help or bring on the menstrual flow.

Monkshood (Aconitum napellus)

Used to treat sciatica and arthritis, measles and nerves related to skin problems, Monkshood is listed as a poisonous plant. Acting as a sedative, an anodyne and

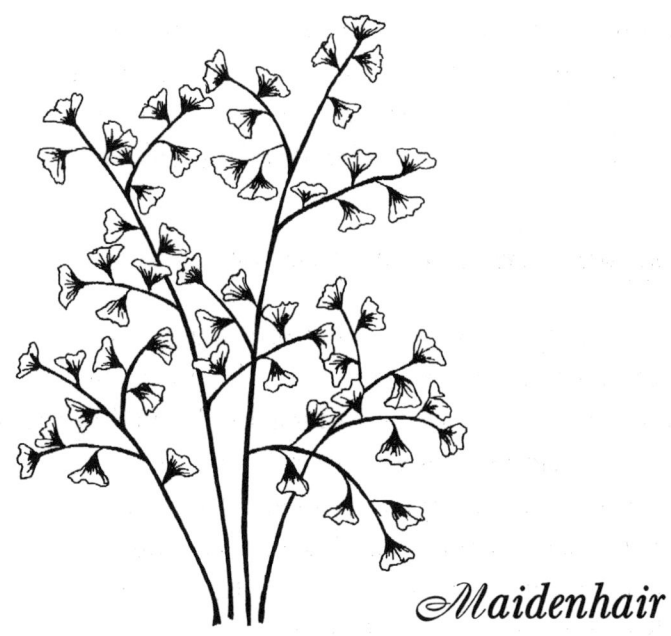

Maidenhair

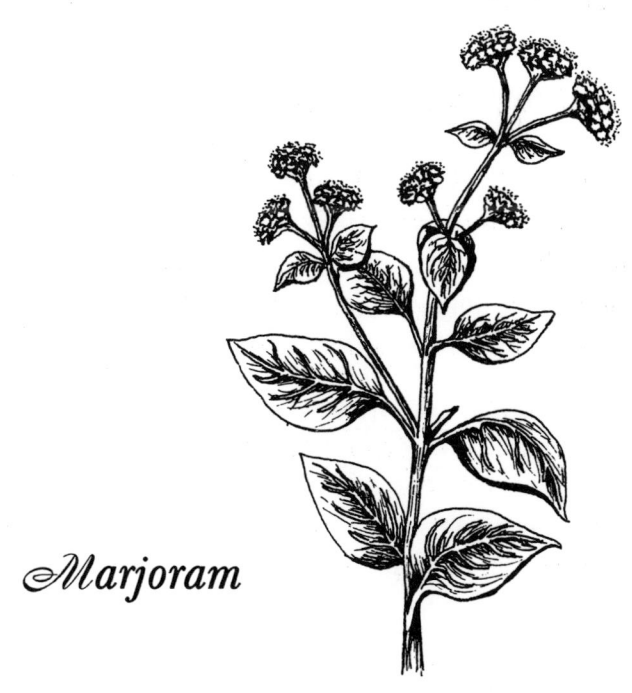

Marjoram

febrifuge, the herb has been known to cure chronic skin problems historically. Its common name is Aconite, and when used by homeopaths can be used to treat a fever.

*WARNING: Even a small dose can cause death.

Motherwort (Leonurus cardiaca)

Its name calls to effect its historical use of bringing joy to the mother by settling the womb and tending to the "vapours," fainting and swooning and "tremblings of the heart." It can be used as a tonic for the heart, to regulate blood pressure during menopause. Motherwort is a sedative and can be used to alleviate anxiety. Motherwort has a good benefit on the stomach and where there is shortness of breath due to anxiety. Motherwort has a similar action to Valerian Root.

Mullein (Verbascum thapsus)

Mullein is historically and in modern times used for lung problems, especially asthma and bronchitis. Historically, it was used to reduce swellings and inflammations, and sinus problems. It has also relieved earache. The fresh flowers are said to remove warts.

Myrrh (Commiphora myrrha)

Used as an astringent, antiseptic, carminative, and a stomachic, Myrrh will relieve a sore mouth and gums,

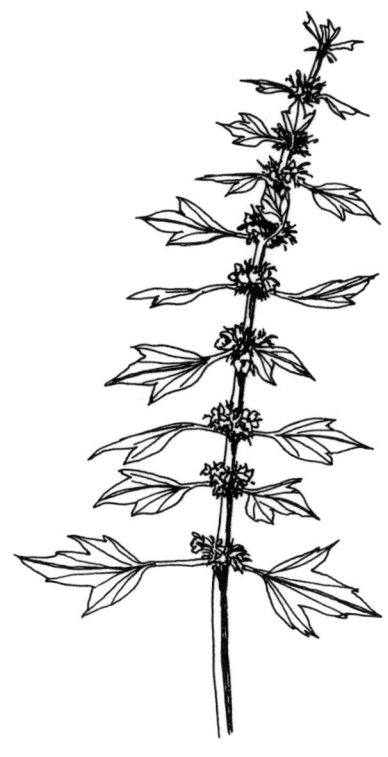

Motherwort

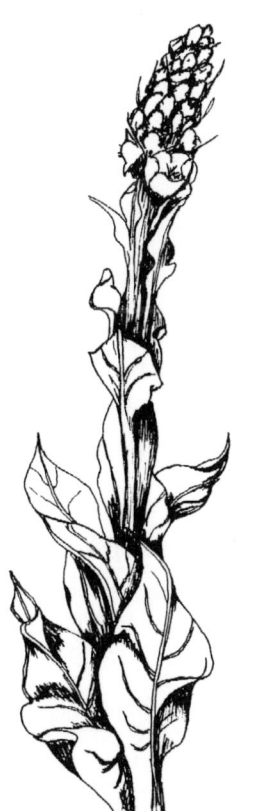

Mullein

asthma, and other chest complaints. Myrrh is a resin that is exuded by trees in Africa and Arabia. It can be made into a powder to treat sores or wounds.

Nettle (Urtica dioica)

The Nettle is an astringent, diuretic, galactagogue, hemostatic, and tonic. It is known as the Stinging Nettle and is actually a perennial growing to about four feet. When touched, the prickly hairs of the plant cause histamine and formic acid to form which produce a sting. The mineral-rich leaves are used to treat anemia and as a blood purifier. Homeopaths use the fresh plant for eczema. Nettles are also helpful for the urinary tract.

*CAUTION: Old Nettle plants should not be eaten as they can cause kidney damage and/or poisoning.

Nutmeg (Myristica fragrans)

This is a tropical fruit native to Indonesia and provides the spice, mace. Nutmeg has been used historically for hundreds of years to treat stomach upset and kidney problems as well. It is an aromatic, too, and has been known to be a mild hallucinogen. Its properties are not unlike marijuana.

*CAUTION: Eating of Nutmeg can cause death or, in smaller doses, stomach pains.

Onion (Allium cepa)

Onion increases the appetite, thirst and increases sperm. It has been known to kill worms in children. It is an antiseptic, diuretic and an expectorant. It acts on coughs and is of benefit to asthma, bronchitis, hayfever and rhinitis. Onion is an excellent internal antiseptic and fights parasites. Research conducted in Czechoslovakia has found Onion to draw bacteria from the air in a sickroom. Onion has been found to lower blood-sugar levels.

Parsley (Petroselinum sativus)

Parsley has been recorded as useful in bladder infections. It can be taken with Echinacea and Marshmallow Root for the treatment of jaundice, asthma, and water retention. Avoid where there is acute infection or inflammation, especially where the kidneys are involved. Parsley acts on the urinary tract and promotes urine. It can comfort the stomach. The root is good for treating diseases of the liver and gallbladder.

Passion Flower (Passiflora incarnata)

Passion Flower acts on the nerves and circulation which brings about sleep, especially after emotional upset. Passion Flower is important for mental worry and over-tiredness. It strengthens the nervous system.

Passion Flower is one of the most exotic flowering vines and is also seen to be symbolic of the crucifixion.

The Passion Flower's ten petals are said to be symbolic of the Apostles. The Cornea symbolizes the Crown of Thorns that was placed on Christ's head, and the five anthers are a symbol of the Five Wounds suffered by Christ. The three stigmas of the Passion Flower symbolize the Three Nails placed in Christ's hands and affixed to his feet holding him to the cross.

Penny Royal (Hedeoma pulegioides)

Historically Penny Royal has been used for fevers and lung infections and drives out heat and inflammation through the pores of the skin. It increases circulation. It has been made with Brewer's Yeast into a tea to bring about abortion. It should not be used by those with a tendency towards excessive menses. American Indians used Penny Royal for headache and for menstrual cramps and pain.

*WARNING: Penny Royal should not be taken during pregnancy.

Peony (Paeonia officinalis)

The Peony is used as a diuretic, sedative and as an antispasmodic. Historically, the Peony has been used for bladder and kidney problems and is an old treatment for jaundice. The Peony is an excellent remedy for epilepsy or spasms and convulsions of any kind. Its results come largely from the root, which is beneficial to the liver.

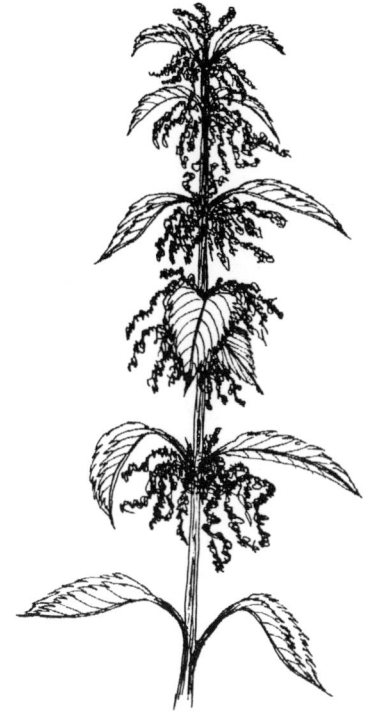

Nettle

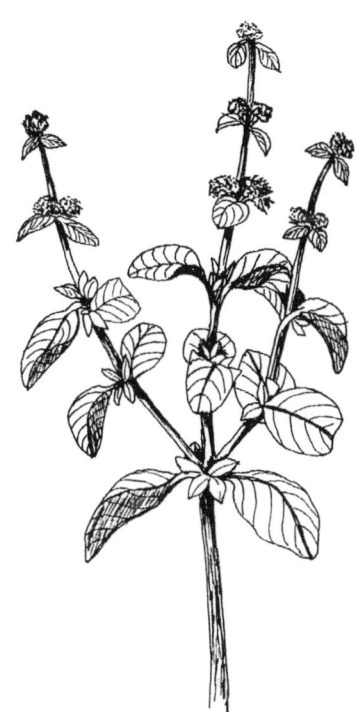

Penny Royal

*Caution: The entire plant is poison and should only be used under professional supervision.

Peppermint (Mentha piperita)

Peppermint acts on the stomach, intestines, muscles and the circulatory system. It is excellent for eliminating nausea, vomiting, chills, colic, fever, gas, diarrhea, and digestive problems. It can be soothing and relaxing.

Plantain (Plantago major)

The Plantain's leaves and roots have been used historically for centuries. Because the Roman Legions found it always under their feet when they needed it in battle, it was known as planta "the sole of man's foot." It treats asthma, earache and kidney disorders. These are only a few ailments Plantain has been known to heal. It has been used for chronic skin diseases due to its richness in potassium salts. It has also been said that Plantain can increase virility.

Poison Hemlock (Conium maculatum)

Dangerously poisonous, the Poison Hemlock has been used historically to execute criminals. The most well-known of its victims being Socrates, Poison Hemlock can sedate and kill if given in the right dosage. Unfortunately, it resembles Anise, and so is sometimes taken in error.

Plantain

Poison Hemlock

Poke Root (Phytolacca decandra-americana)

The roots and the berries of Poke Root can be used medicinally and some herbalists consider Poke Root to be as important as Sarsaparilla as an alterative, meaning having an action on the body that is gradual and nutritive. It can be used for various skin ailments and has been considered as a successful remedy for Psoriasis.

Pomegranate (Punica granatum)

The Pomegranate is an anthelmintic and an astringent. It has been known historically to give relief from tapeworm through use of its seeds. Pomegranate has a high tannin content and so produces a good astringent effect.

Poplar (Populus candicans)

The Balm of Gilead, as this tree is better known, has balsamic properties. It is also a stimulant and an expectorant. As an inhalant, it breaks up congestion from the colds or flu. Poplar acts much like aspirin and can relieve minor aches and pains.

Privet (Ligustrum vulgare)

This plant is an astringent and has bitter properties. Privet can be helpful in cases of diarrhea. Washing the skin with Privet will take away bacteria, and Privet can be

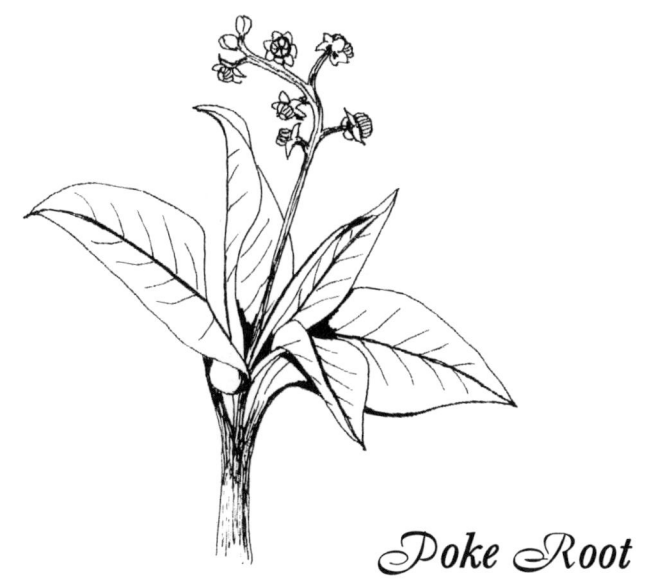

Poke Root

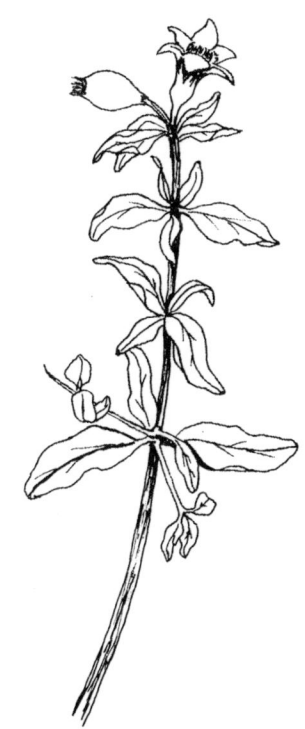

Pomegranate

used as a mouthwash or gargle.

Psyllium Seeds (Plantago ovata)

Psyllium Seeds affect the bowels and intestines and are an excellent cleanser for colitis. They eliminate the toxins in the colon.

Pumpkin (Cucurbita pepo)

Pumpkin is a good treatment for worms. It is an excellent anthelmintic for adults and children. The seed oil has been used for burns and chapped skin.

Rose (Rosa Damascena)

There are many species of rose, but the Damask Rose is of the "old garden" with unknown origins. It grows wild in France and can be made into a syrup with very little effort. By infusing flowers in boiling water and straining, adding sugar, a syrup used for cleaning the colon is produced. The Rose syrup is also beneficial for hemorrhages, and the flowers powdered can stop excessive menstrual bleeding. The Damask Rose as a tincture with dried petals can relieve vomiting and stomach pain.

Rosemary (Rosemarinus officinalis)

Rosemary is good for nervous headaches, tremblings

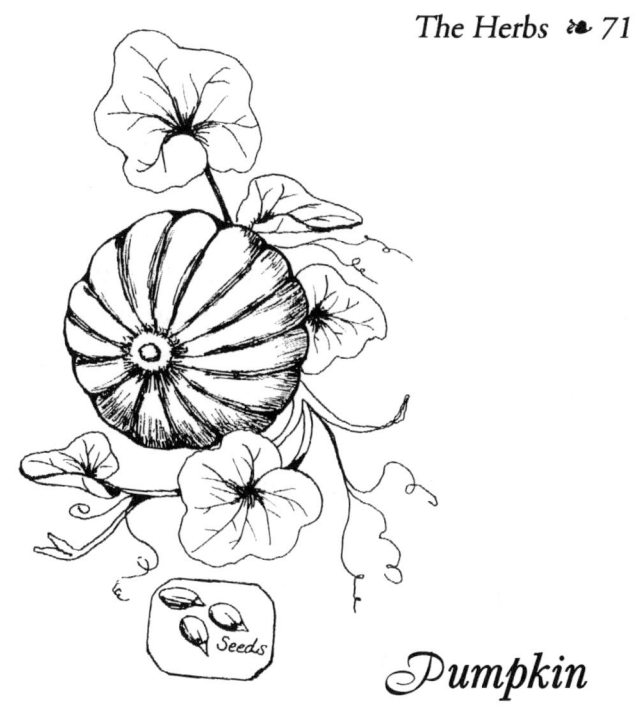

Pumpkin

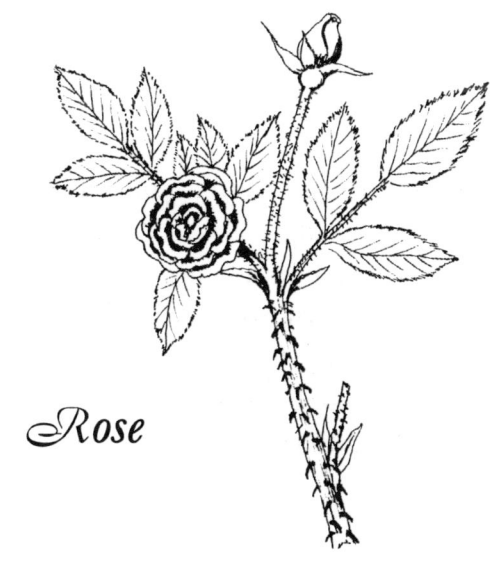

Rose

and other problems related to menopause. It is slightly stimulating and so, therefore, is known as a tonic. Rosemary has been known to cause hallucinations. Rosemary is used as a flavoring for food, and is known historically to promote liver function. Leaves made into a salve can be used against rheumatism, sores, eczema, bruises and old wounds. Rosemary has been known as an excellent hairwash to promote hair growth.

*CAUTION: Excessive amounts of Rosemary taken internally can cause poisoning, or even death.

Safflower (Carthamus tinctorius)

The oil of Safflower is used as a laxative that works on the intestines in a non-irritating way. Safflower lowers cholesterol in the blood stream. It balances the skin, stomach, kidneys, pancreas, nerves and eliminates uric acid. Safflower seeds should not be taken during pregnancy because they are toxic and can cause abortion.

Saffron (Crocus sativus)

Saffron can be used for insomnia, gas, coughs, and to stimulate the appetite. For gout, it relieves pain and swelling through application of a poultice.

It has been known historically to relieve symptoms of hysteric depressions, faintings, and palpitations of the heart. It strengthens the stomach and will expel jaundice.

*CAUTION: Saffron acts as a poison on the central nervous

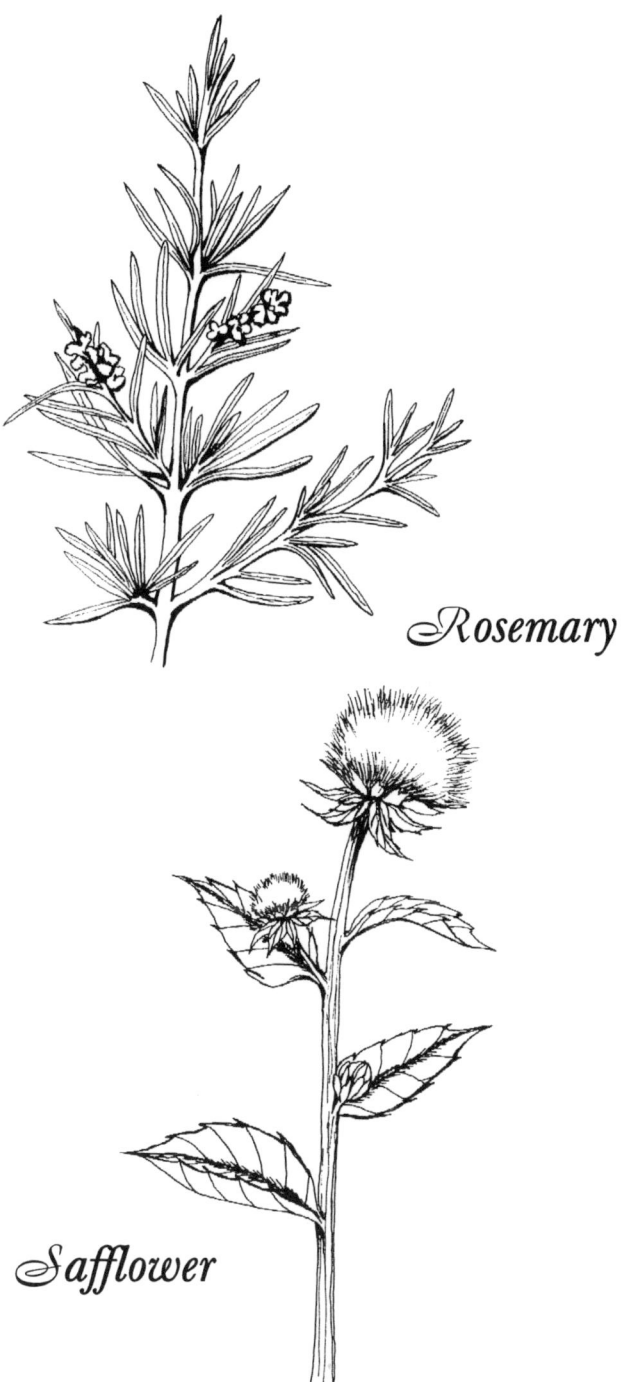

Rosemary

Safflower

system and has been known to cause fatality in humans.

Sage (Salvia officinalis)

Sage has an action on the bowels, sinuses, bladder, mucous membranes and the head and memory. It aids in inflamed gums, and has been known to stop bleeding. Sage is an excellent remedy for flu, diarrhea, indigestion, dysentery, fevers and headaches. Sage is good for the nerves, head and brain. Sage stops lactation, lung congestion, and helps with nausea, night sweats, snake bites, yeast infection and the palsy.

Sandalwood (Santalum album)

Its properties are astringent, disinfectant, diuretic, expectorant, and is also used as a stimulant. The oil can be used for inflammation in mucous tissue, and skin problems have also benefited from Sandalwood. Bacteria is particularly effected by Sandalwood. It is also beneficial in cleansing mentally heavy thoughts or ideas from the mind in preparation for meditation.

Sarsaparilla (Smilax ornata)

Sarsaparilla purifies the urino-genital tract dispelling infection and inflammation. It was used as a Spring Tonic with Yellow Dock. It contains hormone-like substances

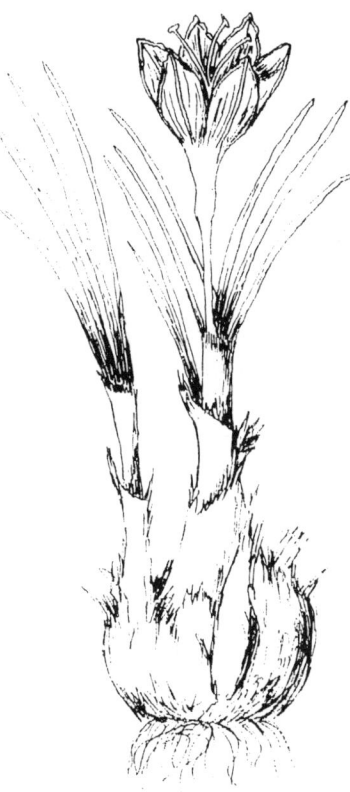

Saffron

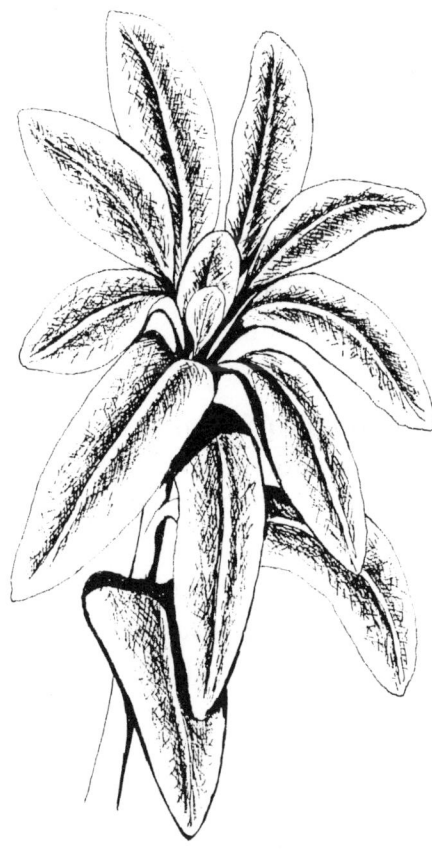

Sage

that externally fight skin parasites. Sarsaparilla has a good action on the blood, skin, circulation and intestines; balances female hormones, and stimulates the body's own immune system. A variety from India has been used to treat syphilis. Sarsaparilla has been used as a treatment for gout, rheumatism, colds, fevers, and even epilepsy. It purifies the blood and increases digestive juices and dispels air from the intestines.

Sassafras (Sassafras officinale)

One of the oldest and most highly recommended remedies of North America, Sassafras was historically used as a Spring Tonic by Native Americans. It is an excellent blood purifier and stimulates the action of the liver to remove toxins from the system.

Sassafras has a good action on the blood for skin disorders, especially acne. It is also a powerful diuretic and can be used for excessive yin conditions. It is high in tannins.

Savory (Satureja hortensis)

A good remedy for stomach and intestinal disorders, Savory makes a tea that will counteract nausea and stimulate appetite. It acts as an astringent, and so the tea is a good gargle for a sore throat.

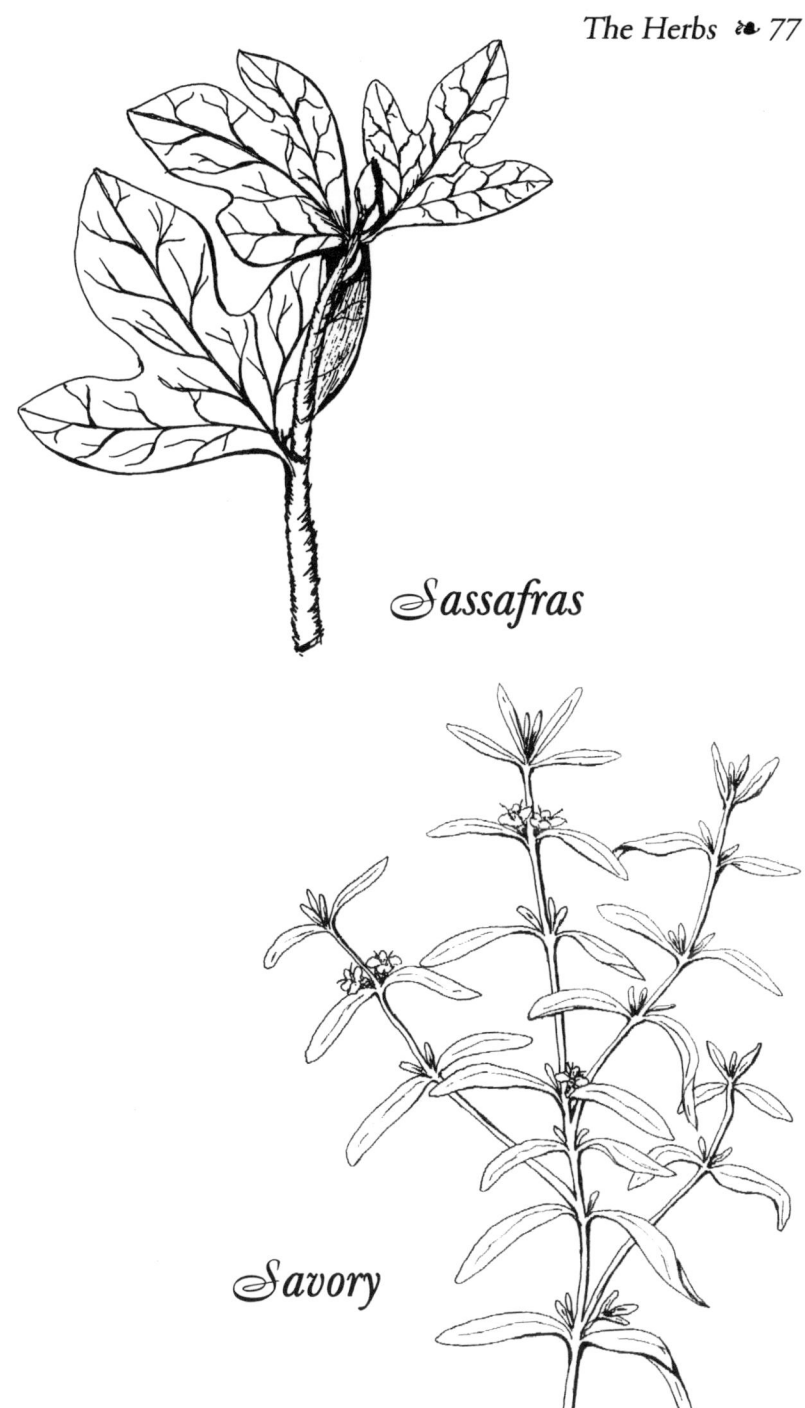

Sassafras

Savory

Saw Palmetto (Serenoa serrulata)

Used in modern times as a method for treating prostate problems, Saw Palmetto berries are useful for asthma and bronchitis as well. Known to strengthen glandular tissue, Saw Palmetto has also been considered to possess aphrodisiac powers.

Senna (Cassia acutifolia)

One of the most powerful laxatives, Senna needs to be combined with a carminative, which is an agent for dispelling gas. Such an herb would be Ginger, Cardamom, Coriander or Fennel. This would prevent bowel cramps. The pods of Senna have a milder action than the leaves.

Sesame Seeds (Sesamum indicum)

Sesame Seeds are good for respiration, weak lungs and for constipation. They have been known to heal tissue and stop tooth decay. Sesame Seeds help constipation and hemorrhoids, and they treat hair loss and receding gums. They are good for the feet. Sesame Seeds are used for lightness to help in higher and clearer meditations.

Skullcap (Scutellaria lateriflora)

Historically, Skullcap has been used to treat nerves and

the stomach. It has a good action on digestive problems and emotional problems leading to worry. The American Indians used Skullcap to promote the menses and were said to have cured rabies with it. It has been used successfully with alcoholics to treat delirium tremens.

Slippery Elm (Ulmus fulva)

Slippery Elm is beneficial for the whole body. It strengthens and heals and soothes inflamed or irritated areas and absorbs noxious gases. Slippery Elm is used to neutralize stomach acidity.

Sorrel (Rumex acetosa)

This is Common Sorrel and historically was known to quench thirst and bring on the appetite. It is a cooling herb, and so can be used for inflammations of all kinds, especially those originating in the blood. It is eaten in salads and will sharpen the taste. It contains oxalic acid which cannot be tolerated by people with rheumatic conditions. Sorrel can also be used as a laxative, and the root has been used to treat external skin irritations such as eczema and acne.

Tarragon (Artemisia dracunculus)

Tarragon is a diuretic used to stimulate the kidneys and is used as a drying agent. By using only the young tops, Tarragon will bring on the menses. Tarragon stimulates the appetite and the digestion. Tarragon Tea at bedtime is a remedy for sleeplessness due to its hypnotic properties.

Thyme (Thymus vulgaris)

Thyme has historically been used to aid in bronchitis, whooping cough, diarrhea, gas and lack of appetite. Thyme has been used with success in athletes foot and to remove skin parasites. Cooking with Thyme has a good action on the lungs. Oil of Thyme can be used for its antiseptic action for a mouthwash or gargle.

*WARNING: Excessive use of Thyme can over stimulate the thyroid gland and will result in poisoning.

Turmeric (Curcuma longa)

Turmeric is a good blood purifier and stimulant. It breaks up congestion. In India it is referred to as the Divine Mother or the Grandmother. It is used with Almond and Sesame oil for an external rub. Turmeric is a main ingredient in curry.

Valerian (Valerian officinalis)

Valerian is sedating and calming to the emotions. It is a nervine, which means it treats and nourishes the nerves. It is soothing to the nervous system and helps reduce anxiety,

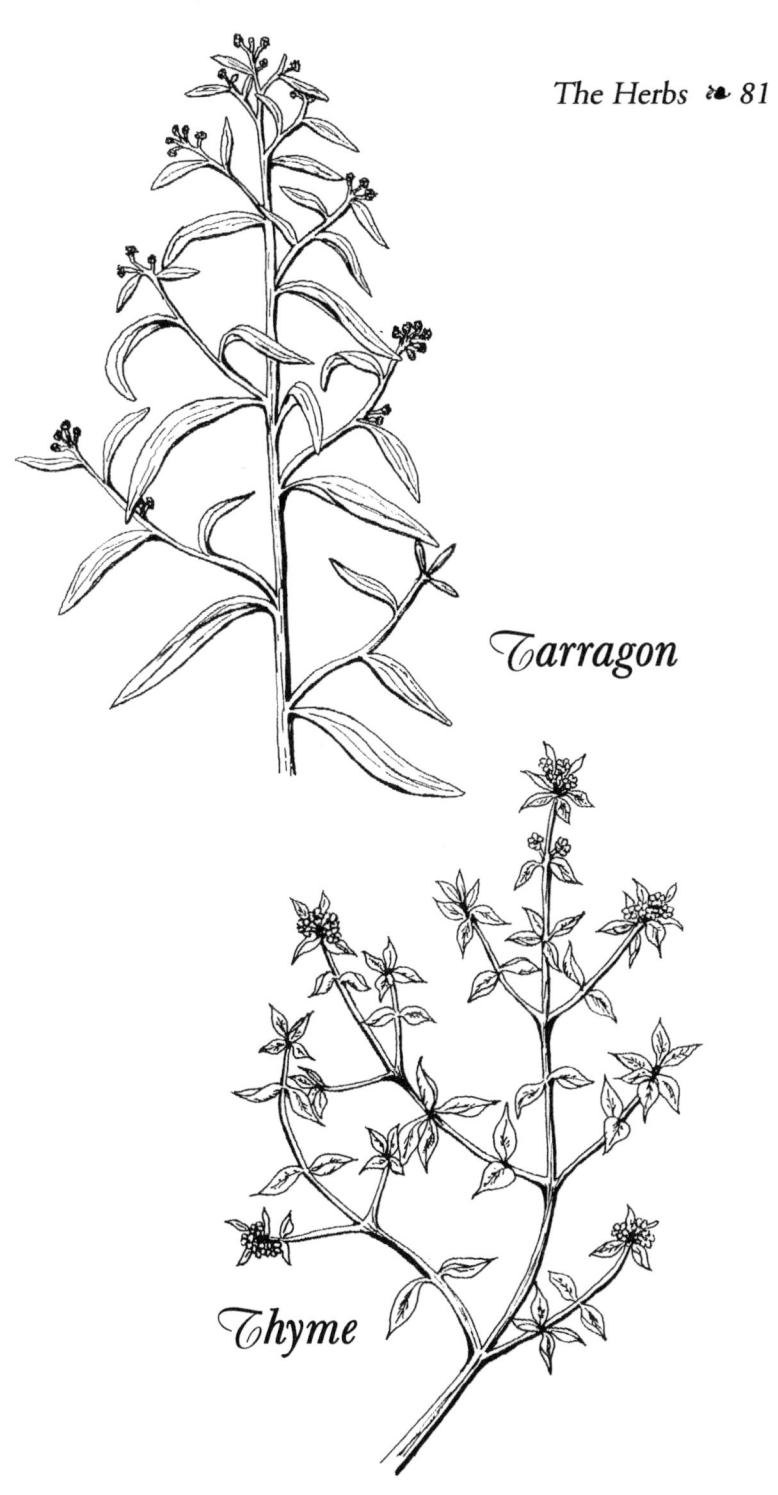

Tarragon

Thyme

tension and hysteria. It eases pain and promotes sleep with no damaging side-effects.

White Pine (Pinus strobus)

Native Americans used White Pine's inner bark as a remedy for congestion. Some used the sap along with the leaves as a cold treatment. It was recorded from many Native American tribes that the inner bark or the sap could be used externally on wounds.

Willow (Salix alba)

Willow properties are antiseptic and astringent. The Willow is also a diuretic, diaphoretic, febrifuge and a tonic. It is also an anodyne. Willow's main function is to relieve pain and to reduce fever. It contains salicin which is changed to salicylic acid in the body. Willow Bark reduces inflammation and has been used for thousands of years. It is particularly effective as a diuretic for rheumatism and gout and is also good for the stomach. Externally, Willow Bark washes burns and wounds and eruptions with a good effect.

Witch Hazel (Hamamelis virginiana)

Used as an astringent, a sedative and a tonic, Witch Hazel has been used for skin irritations for centuries. It is best known for its astringent properties, but has also been

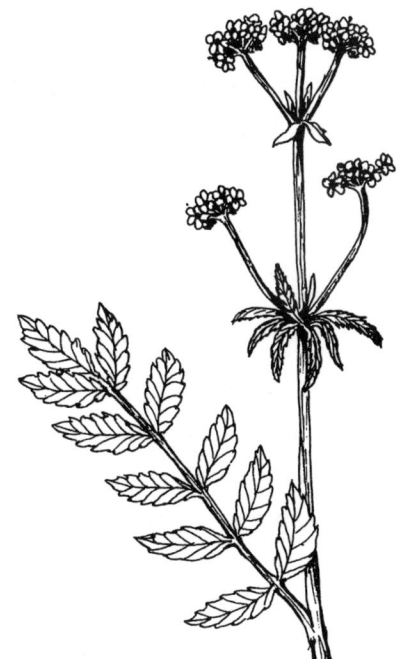

Valerian

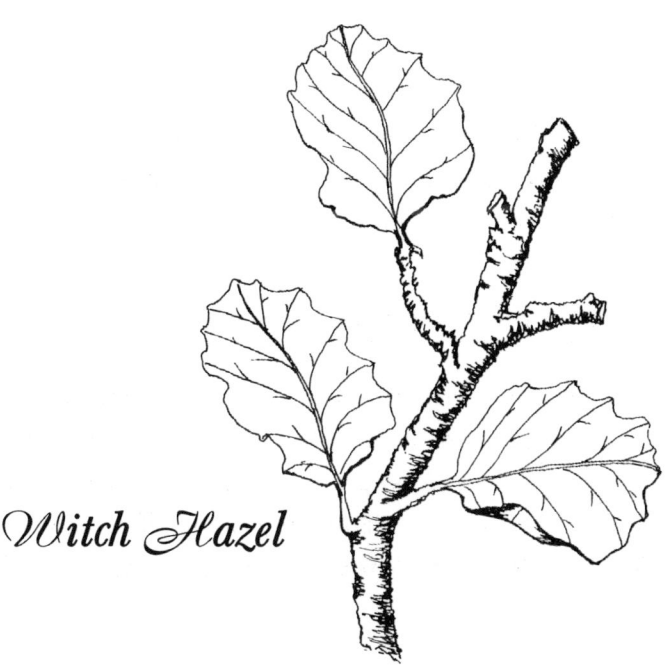

Witch Hazel

known to remedy eye inflammation and hemorrhoids owing to its sedative and hemostatic properties. The inner bark can be made into a poultice for this job.

Wormwood (Artemisia absinthium)

The name usually used for Wormwood is Absinthe. Wormwood is an anthelmintic, an antiseptic, an antispasmodic, carminative, cholagogue, febrifuge, stimulant and a stomachic. It has an excellent benefit to the stomach, treating gas pain and a lack of appetite. Historically, it has been known to treat the liver by stimulating it. The oil acts to relieve pain of rheumatism and arthritis. Wormwood can improve circulation and has a good effect on heat.

Yarrow (Achillea millefolium)

Yarrow is a cooling herb and acts as an astringent. It reduces fire and excess bile and inflammation. It has historically been used for kidney infection.

Yellow Dock (Rumex crispus)

Known as an astringent and a tonic, Yellow Dock has been used as a medicinal plant since very ancient times. It was known as a blood purifier and fought eruptive diseases and other skin problems very well. The leaves of the Yellow Dock were used to remedy boils by Native

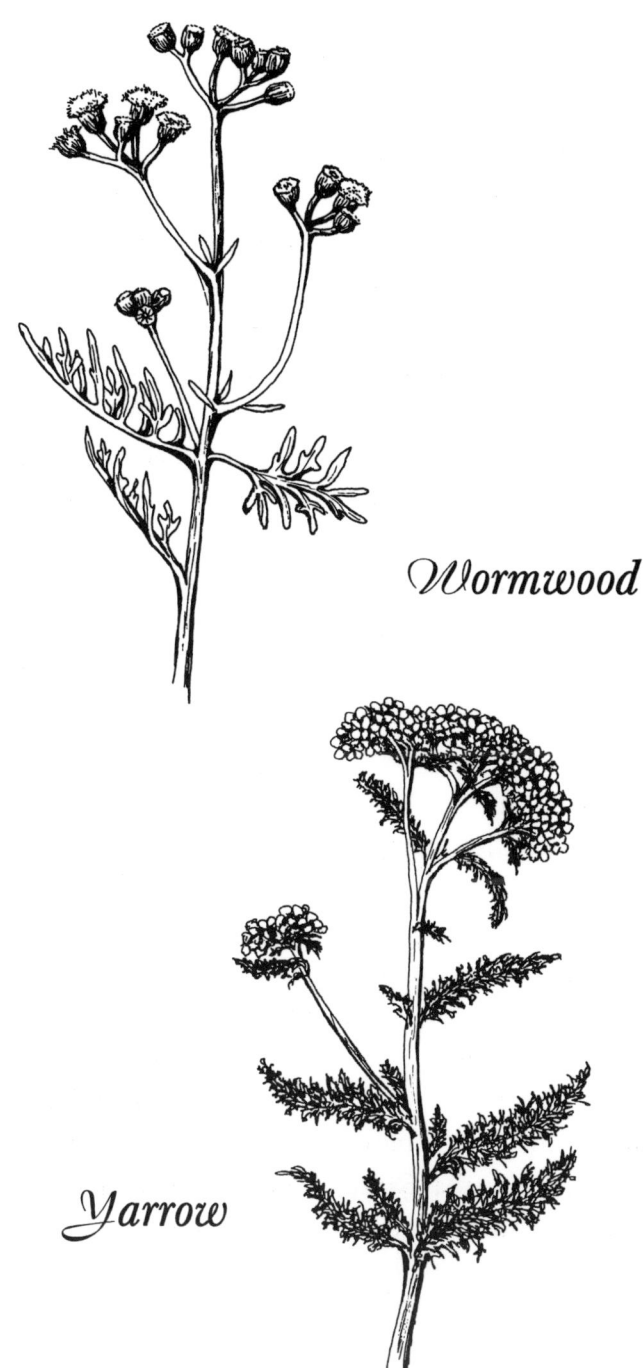

Wormwood

Yarrow

Americans, and the root was applied to cuts to dry the wound. Because it is rich in Vitamin A, Yellow Dock can fight problems with the Liver and will remedy bleeding in the Lungs. Leprosy is one of the diseases historically listed that Yellow Dock has had proven results with. Rheumatism, stomach problems, thyroid problems and glands are all benefited by Yellow Dock.

Yellow Gentian (Gentiana lutea)

The properties of this herb are cholagogue, febrifuge, refrigerant, tonic, and stomachic. Yellow Gentian increases the appetite and helps strengthen the stomach. It has been used successfully in indigestion, diarrhea and vomiting; also in cases of fainting spells. It has been used externally for a wound wash. Because Yellow Gentian is a refrigerant, it has a good effect on inflamed or irritated tissue.

Yerba Santa (Eriodictyon californicum)

Yerba Santa is an antispasmodic, an expectorant, febrifuge and a tonic. It is known to be an excellent expectorant. Used largely to treat bronchitis, lung problems and asthma, it has been known as a blood purifier since the early 1800's. Native Americans use Yerba Santa for asthma by smoking it or chewing the leaves. Externally, Yerba Santa is important as a poultice for bruises, wounds, and any kind of insect bite.

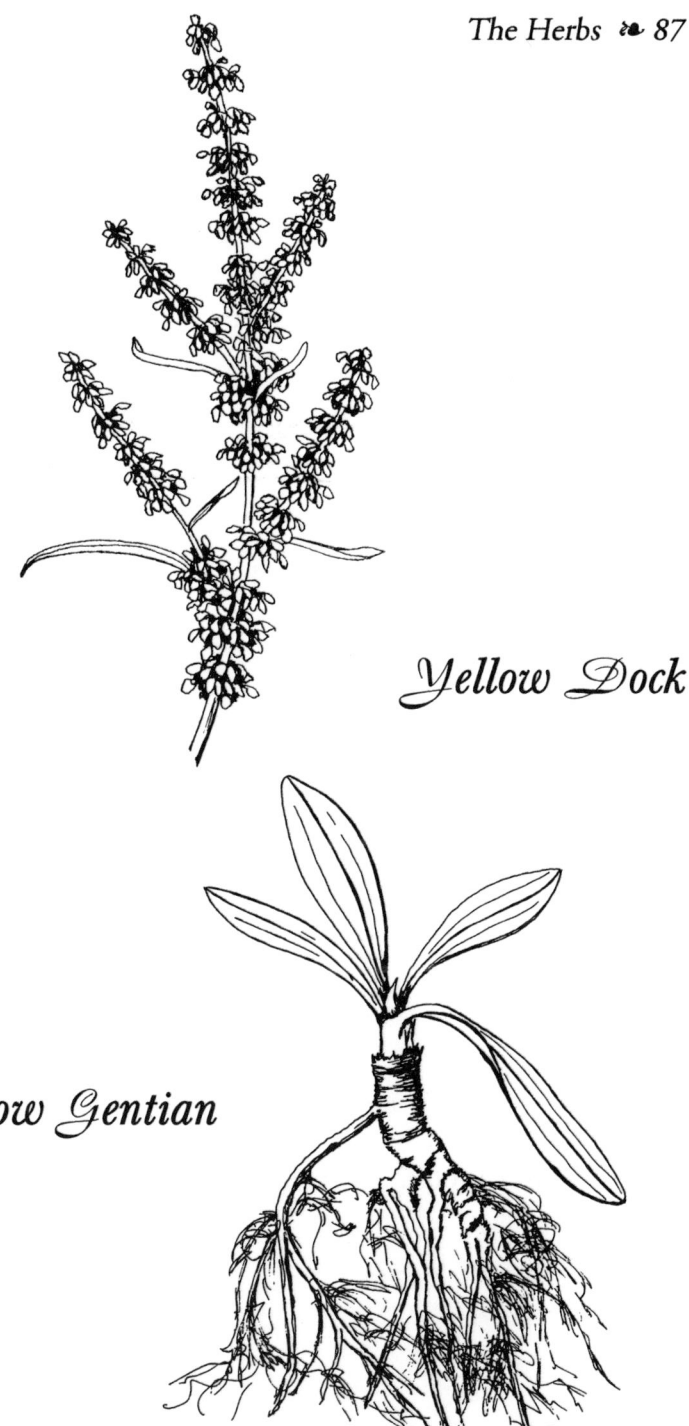

Yellow Dock

Yellow Gentian

Ways Herbs Can Be Prepared

Infusion -- Tea

To properly use the volatile oils of herbs, boil water and pour the boiling water over the herb, steeping for two to eight minutes. Strain through the leaves or flowers used to prepare the tea. Do not boil the actual herb itself but let the herb steep in boiled water until desired strength of herbal tea has been achieved.

Another method of infusion is to use the sun's rays to heat the herbs in water. Use a glass jar with a tight lid and expose to the sun for a few hours.

Decoction--Tea

To get the deeper essences from the herbs, simmer the herb in an uncovered pot for about an hour, until about 1/3 or 1/2 of the water has evaporated. To get to coarser herbs such as Valerian, Cinnamon and Burdock Root simmer about an hour in a covered pot. Always strain before using.

Fomentation—External

To externally treat with herbs, for example swellings, pains and even colds, prepare a soaking towel or cloth saturated with the herbal tea. The towel should be hot and placed over the area of affliction without burning the skin. Sometimes placing a dry cloth over the wet one helps to lock the vapors into the wound.

Poultice—External

To apply herbs directly over the skin, is referred to as a poultice. To make a poultice, add water to the powdered or macerated herb until a thick paste forms. Then apply the warm paste directly onto the skin. This method is good for pulling out infection and relieving swelling or inflammation.

Plaster—External

If an area needs treatment but cannot be touched with the direct application of the herb, place the herb between two pieces of cloth, linen or cotton. Make sure the cloth is pleasing to the skin and can properly contain the herbs, but also allow them to send their vapors to the area of application.

Salve—External

To make a salve, first make an herbal oil, adding unmelted beeswax. Extract the herbs in hot oil, allowing two hours for roots and barks to extract the oil by heating just below boiling. Leaves and flowers will take under an hour to be extracted. Roots will take longer to produce the oils needed for a salve.

Use two ounces of the herb to six ounces of vegetable shortening and one ounce of beeswax. The substance will become cold, producing a salve that is firm to the touch. Then it is ready to be applied to the afflicted area.

Extract--Internal

For those people who cannot swallow capsules or pills of any kind, add herbal liquid to water which produces an extract and can be taken internally.

Capsules--Internal

Powdered herbs should be placed in a gelatin capsule, readily available at health food stores. This method is the easiest to ingest for some people and produces an easy and exact dosage.

Tinctures--Internal

To keep concentrated forms of herbal extract for long periods of time, add the herbal extract to an alcohol base. The alcohol is used as a preservative. This form of herbal application will further concentrate the properties of the herb, in that the alcohol itself will draw out the ingredients of the herb. Combine three to four ounces of an herb with one pint of brandy, gin, vodka or rum. Let it sit for two weeks. Let the herbs settle and pour off the tincture that forms. Strain out all unwanted materials.

Cleansing Program

Juicing is a program that <u>adds</u> to an already good dietary plan. All juices can stimulate the digestive tract, and are important for cleansing. Taken along with solid food diets, juices help balance and promote healing.

<u>Vegetable and Fruit Juices for Cleansing</u>

8 ounces Carrot Juice / 2 ounces Celery Juice / 1 ounce Lemon Juice

7 ounces Cucumber Juice / 2 ounces Endive Juice / 1/2 ounce Pineapple Juice

8 ounces Aloe Vera Juice 1 x daily, especially in the morning

4 ounces Celery Juice 3 x daily.

4 ounces Parsley Juice 2 x daily.

8 ounces Carrot Juice 3 x daily.

4 ounces Apple Juice 3 x daily.

4 ounces Pineapple Juice 4 x daily.

8 ounces Black Cherry Juice 2 x daily.

<u>Herbs for Cleansing</u>

Dandelion
Dong Quai
Ginseng
Golden Seal

Common Name Index

A Few Sources for Easy Reference and Further Study of Herbs

Back to Eden, Jethro Kloss.

A Barefoot Doctor's Manual, The American Translation of the *Official Chinese Paramedical Manual*.

Common Herbs for Common Illnesses, William R. McGrath, N.D.

Essential Oils that Build Natural Defenses, The Science of Aromatherapy, Dr. William H. Lee with Greg Holt, Biochemist.

Folk Medicine, D.C. Jarvis, M.D.

Healing With Herbs and Vitamins, Dr. Samuels Troyer, D.C.

Health Handbook, Louise Tenney M.H.

The Herb Book, John Lust, N.D.

Herbal Healing by Michael Hallowell.

The Herbalist Almanac, Indiana Botanical Gardens, 1954.

Indian Doctor Book, Compiled and Published by Nancy Locke Doane.

Just Weeds, Pamela Jones

Los Remedios de la Gente, Compiled by Michael Moore.

Medicinal Plants of the Mountain West, by Michael Moore.

The Medicine Show, by the Editors of *Consumer Reports.*

Natural Herbal Formulas, Dr. Stan Malstrom, N.D., M.D.

Prescription for Nutritional Healing, James F. Balch, C.N.C.

Seven Herbs, Plants and Teachers, Matthew Wood

The Simmonite-Culpeper Herbal Remedies, Dr. W.J. Simmonite and Nicolas Culpeper

The Way of Herbs, Michael Tierra, C.A., N.D.

The Yoga of Herbs by Dr. Vasant Lad and David Frawley.

Editor's Note

Mary Ann Dykes has had experience in the Natural Healing Education field for the past 16 years. She is the founder and director of

Heartway Healing Center®

a natural healing education center.

located in New Orleans and LaCombe, Louisiana. She is a naturalist, writer, and photographer.